MRI of the Brain I

Second Edition

The LWW MRI Teaching File Series

SERIES EDITORS

Robert B. Lufkin
William G. Bradley, Jr.
Michael Brant-Zawadzki

MRI of the Brain I

William G. Bradley, Jr., Michael Brant-Zawadzki, and Jane Cambray-Forker

MRI of the Brain II

Michael Brant-Zawadzki, Jane Cambray-Forker, and William G. Bradley, Jr.

MRI of the Spine

Jeffrey S. Ross

MRI of the Head and Neck

Robert B. Lufkin, Alexandra Borges, Kim N. Nguyen, and Yoshimi Anzai

MRI of the Musculoskeletal System

Karence K. Chan and Mini Pathria

Pediatric MRI

Rosalind B. Dietrich

The LWW MRI Teaching File Series

MRI of the Brain I

Second Edition

Editors

William G. Bradley, Jr., M.D., Ph.D.
Director, MRI and Radiology Research
Department of Radiology
Long Beach Memorial Medical Center
Long Beach, California

Professor
Department of Radiological Sciences
University of California, Irvine
Orange, California

Michael Brant-Zawadzki, M.D.
Medical Director
Department of Radiology
Hoag Memorial Hospital Presbyterian
Newport Beach, California

Clinical Professor of Diagnostic Radiology
Stanford University
Stanford, California

Jane Cambray-Forker, D.O.
Director, Spinal Imaging
Department of Radiology
St. Joseph's Hospital
Orange, California

Assistant Clinical Professor
Department of Diagnostic Radiology
University of California, Irvine
College of Medicine
Orange, California

Associate Editors

Peter Brotchie, M.B.B.S., Ph.D.
Director of MRI
The Geelong Hospital
Geelong, Victoria, Australia

Sattam Saud Lingawi, M.D.
The University Hospital
King Abdulaziz University
Jeddah, Saudi Arabia

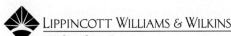
LIPPINCOTT WILLIAMS & WILKINS
A **Wolters Kluwer** Company
Philadelphia • Baltimore • New York • London
Buenos Aires • Hong Kong • Sydney • Tokyo

Acquisitions Editor: Joyce-Rachel John
Developmental Editor: Denise Martin
Production Editor: Maria Tortora
Manufacturing Manager: Tim Reynolds
Cover Designer: Jeane Norton
Compositor: Maryland Composition
Printer: Maple Press

© 2001 by LIPPINCOTT WILLIAMS & WILKINS
530 Walnut Street
Philadelphia, PA 19106 USA
LWW. com

Printed in the USA

Library of Congress Cataloging-in-Publication Data

MRI of the Brain I / editors, William G. Bradley, Jr., Michael Brant-Zawadzki, Jane Cambray-Forker; associate editors, Peter Brotchie, Sattam Saud Lingawi.— 2nd ed.
    p. ; cm. — (The LWW MRI teaching file series)
  Rev. ed. of: MRI of the brain. New York : Raven press, c1991.
  Includes bibliographical references and index.
  ISBN 0-7817-2569-0 (Volume 1)
  ISBN 0-7817-2568-2 (Volume 2)
    1. Brain—Magnetic resonance imaging. 2. Brain—Diseases—Diagnosis. I. Bradley, William G. II. Brant-Zawadzki, Michael. III. Cambray-Forker, Jane. IV. MRI of the brain. V. Series.
    [DNLM: 1. Brain Diseases—diagnosis. 2. Magnetic Resonance Imaging. WL 348 B8128 2000]
RC386.6.M34 B74 2000
616.8'047548–dc21

00-061099

Care has been taken to confirm the accuracy of the information presented and to describe generally accepted practices. However, the editors and publisher are not responsible for errors or omissions or for any consequences from application of the information in this book and make no warranty, expressed or implied, with respect to the currency, completeness, or accuracy of the contents of the publication. Application of this information in a particular situation remains the professional responsibility of the practitioner.

The editors and publisher have exerted every effort to ensure that drug selection and dosage set forth in this text are in accordance with current recommendations and practice at the time of publication. However, in view of ongoing research, changes in government regulations, and the constant flow of information relating to drug therapy and drug reactions, the reader is urged to check the package insert for each drug for any change in indications and dosage and for added warnings and precautions. This is particularly important when the recommended agent is a new or infrequently employed drug.

Some drugs and medical devices presented in this publication have Food and Drug Administration (FDA) clearance for limited use in restricted research settings. It is the responsibility of the health care provider to ascertain the FDA status of each drug or device planned for use in their clinical practice.

10 9 8 7 6 5 4 3 2 1

*Although we do not want to take anything away
from our wives, children, mentors, or students,
this volume is dedicated to the neurosis which
results in our writing books when
we could be playing golf or going fishing.*

*W. G. B.
M. B.-Z.*

*To my husband, Gerry, for his unwavering support, encouragement, and faith in me.
To my children, Britton and Shane, who make everything worthwhile.
To my teachers, mentors, and friends,
Drs. Michael Huckman, Glenn Geremia, and William Greenlee.*

*I would like to give special thanks to Robyn Francis for all her hard work—
I couldn't have done it without you!
Thank you to Dr. Michael Brant-Zawadzki for your help, guidance, and support.
Thanks to all at Irvine Imaging Services.*

J. C.-F.

CONTENTS

Note: Unless otherwise indicated, all cases have been submitted by Jane Cambray-Forker, D.O. and Michael Brant-Zawadzki, M.D., Hoag Memorial Hospital, Newport Beach, California.

PREFACE

Twelve years ago, we approached Mary Rogers, then the president of Raven Press (now Lippincott Williams & Wilkins) to do a 1,000-case, 10-volume MR Teaching File. The fact that they asked us to do it again means it must have been successful. This volume is one of two volumes on the brain and again is edited by us with major contributions from Drs. Cambray, Lingawi, and Brotchie. To preserve the concept of a teaching file, the cases are essentially in random order without grouping by category. This allows the reader to first view the images and read the clinical history followed by the diagnosis and discussion. The discussion has been kept intentionally brief to allow coverage of multiple cases in a short period of time. References are provided for additional reading. As the reader will see, the latest in MR technology—echo planar diffusion, echo planar perfusion, and spectroscopy—are included in this volume. Comparison with the first edition published 10 years ago gives even the most casual observer a good concept of how far we have come in the clinical application of MRI technology. We hope you enjoy reading this teaching file as much as we enjoyed putting it together.

A few people deserve special thanks for this volume including the 1999–2000 MR Fellows at Long Beach Memorial Medical Center, Dr. Sandy Patel (MR Fellow 1997–98), and several residents from the University of California at Irvine who rotated through during the year. Dr. Cambray-Forker at Hoag Memorial Hospital was the major force behind almost all of the content contributed from Hoag and Robyn Francis was an invaluable assistant. We would also like to thank Jim Ryan at Lippincott Williams & Wilkins who persisted in his efforts to put together this second edition and Joyce-Rachel John whose persistence resulted in our completing this project in a timely fashion.

William G. Bradley, Jr., M.D., Ph.D.
Michael Brant-Zawadzki, M.D.

MRI of the Brain I

Second Edition

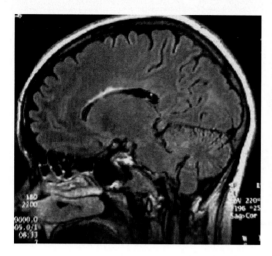
FIG. 1.1A

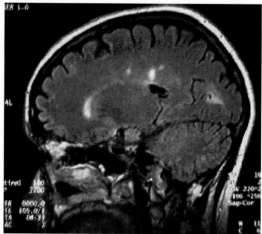
FIG. 1.1B

CLINICAL HISTORY

A 32-year-old woman with clinical history of optic neuritis.

FINDINGS

Hyperintense striations are seen perpendicular to the undersurface of the corpus callosum on the sagittal fluid-attenuated inversion-recovery (FLAIR) image (Fig. 1.1A). Ovoid hyperintense foci are also present in the corona radiata on the parasagittal FLAIR image (Fig. 1.1B). *Submitted by Peter Brotchie, M.B.B.S., Ph.D., Sattam Lingawi, M.B., Ch.B., F.R.C.P.C., and William G. Bradley, M.D., Ph.D., F.A.C.R., Senior Editor, Long Beach Memorial Medical Center, Long Beach, California.*

DIAGNOSIS

Multiple sclerosis (MS).

DISCUSSION

MS is the most common demyelinating disease in countries with temperate climates. It is diagnosed on the basis of recurrent attacks of focal neurological deficits of variable severity involving multiple anatomically unrelated parts of the body. The disease has a multiphasic remitting and relapsing pattern with predilection for the spinal cord, optic nerves, and the periventricular white matter.

MRI is the imaging modality of choice for patients with suspected MS. The disease most often results in high signal intensity foci within the corpus callosum, periventricular white matter, and middle cerebellar peduncles. Although posterior fossa and cord involvement is less frequent, it is more specific. Demyelinating lesions surround the veins, which results in their perpendicular orientation to the ventricular system (histologic "Dawson's fingers"). These are best seen on proton density and fluid attenuated inversion recovery (FLAIR) sequences. T2-weighted images are less reliable for the detection of the periventricular lesions due to partial volume averaging of the hypertense cerebrospinal fluid (however, T2-weighted images are superior to other sequences for detection of lesions in the cord). Thin-section sagittal FLAIR imaging is very sensitive for the detection of subcallosal striations, which are believed to represent the earliest sign of periventricular demyelination. (Subcallosal striations are not easily seen on routine axial magnetic resonance images.)

The primary disease in the differential diagnosis is a monophasic demyelinating process called "acute disseminated encephalomyelitis."

SUGGESTED READING

Palmer S, Bradley WG, Chen D, et al. Subcallosal striations: early findings of multiple sclerosis on sagittal, thin-section, fast FLAIR MR imaging. *Radiology* 1999;210:149–153.

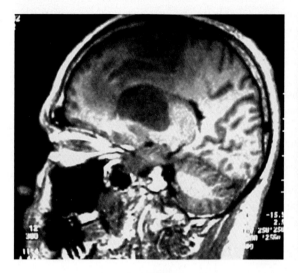

FIG. 2.1A

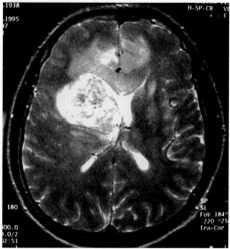

FIG. 2.1B

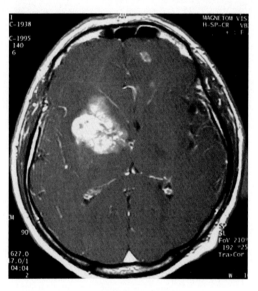

FIG. 2.1C

CLINICAL HISTORY

A 57-year-old man with headaches and recent personality change.

FINDINGS

Right parasagittal T1-weighted image (Fig. 2.1A) demonstrates a large well-defined lesion with low signal in the region of the right basal ganglia. Additionally, there is poorly defined low signal within the posterior right frontal lobe. Axial fast spin echo T2-weighted image (Fig. 2.1B) shows a heterogeneous lesion with predominately high signal, centered within the right basal ganglia. There is associated mass effect with effacement of the right lateral ventricle and shift of the midline structures to the left. Additionally, there is abnormal high signal within the subcortical white matter of the right frontal lobe extending through the corpus callosum into the left frontal lobe. Multifocal enhancement corresponding to the lesions is seen on the postcontrast T1-weighted acquisition (Fig. 2.1C).

DIAGNOSIS

Multicentric glioma.

DISCUSSION

This case helps illustrate the nonspecificity of multifocal enhancing lesions on T1-weighted postcontrast imaging. The typical causes of multiple enhancing foci are metastatic disease and multifocal infection. Vasculitis and multiple emboli are less common causes. Multicentric glioma can simulate these entities when dedifferentiation into more aggressive histologies occurs within a single tumor at separate locations within the lesion.

The pattern of vasogenic edema can help in the differential diagnosis. Vasogenic edema tends to be more extensive in the other entities, with resultant greater mass effect as compared to multicentric primary glioma of the brain. Also, extension of vasogenic edema across the corpus callosum is almost never seen due to the heavily myelinated white matter tracts of the corpus callosum restricting the size of the extracellular space, not allowing extension of vasogenic edema. On the other hand, tumor infiltration through these tracts in cases of glioma is not uncommon.

SUGGESTED READING

Dean BL, Drayer BP, Bird CR, et al. Gliomas: classification with MR imaging. *Radiology* 1990;174:411–415.

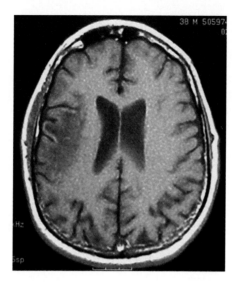

FIG. 3.1A

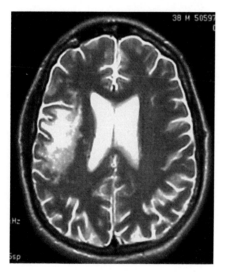

FIG. 3.1B

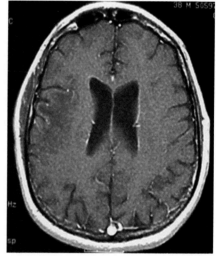

FIG. 3.1C

CLINICAL HISTORY

A 38-year-old man with history of mental status change.

FINDINGS

There is a large region of signal abnormality within the subcortical white matter of the right posterior frontal and parietal lobes, which is characterized by low signal on T1-weighted images and high signal on the fast spin echo T2-weighted images (Fig. 3.1A and B). Postcontrast T1-weighted acquisition (Fig. 3.1C) shows no abnormal enhancement.

DIAGNOSIS

Progressive multifocal leukoencephalopathy (PML).

DISCUSSION

PML is a demyelination disease with a viral etiology. It is the result of the reactivation of the papovavirus (JC type), primarily in the immunocompromised population. One percent to seven percent of the population with acquired immunodeficiency syndrome acquires this universally fatal disease (usually within 6 to 12 months of diagnosis). The disease classically presents as asymmetric bilateral patchy regions of demyelination with preference for the subcortical white matter of the parietooccipital lobes. On imaging, the lesions are low signal on T1-weighted images and high signal on proton density and T2-weighted acquisitions. The gray matter can be involved but is not as noticeable. The corpus callosum, brainstem, and basal ganglia can be involved. There is usually no mass effect, although it has been reported. Hemorrhage and enhancement are extremely uncommon. Differential diagnostic possibilities include cytomegalovirus, human immunodeficiency virus encephalopathy (more commonly confluent, symmetric bilateral periventricular white matter involvement, as opposed to patchy subcortical disease), lymphoma, and glioma (mass effect more common). Thallium-201 single proton emission computed tomography studies can help differentiate PML from tumor, as PML typically does not demonstrate uptake and tumor does; however, there is a recent case report that describes thallium-201 uptake in pathologically proven PML.

SUGGESTED READING

Mark AS, Atlas SW. Progressive multifocal leukoencephalopathy in patients with AIDS: appearance on MRI images. *Radiology* 1989;173(2):517–520.

Port JD, Miseljic S, Lee RR. Progressive multifocal leukoencephalopathy demonstrating contrast enhancement on MRI and uptake of thallium-201: case report. *Neuroradiology* 1999;41(12):895–898.

Rovira MJ, Post MJD, Bowen BC. Central nervous system infections in HIV-infected persons. *Neuroimaging Clin North Am* 1991;1:179–200.

Trotot PM, Vazeaux R, Yamashita HK, et al. MRI patterns of progressive multifocal leukoencephalopathy (PML) in AIDS. Pathologic correlation. *J Neuroradiol* 1990;17(4):233–254.

Whiteman ML, Post MJ, Berger JR, et al. Progressive multifocal leukoencephalopathy in 47 HIV-seropositive patients: neuroimaging with clinical and pathologic correlation. *Radiology* 1993;187(1):233–240.

Woo HH, Rezai AR, Kopp EA, et al. Contrast enhancing progressive multifocal leukoencephalopathy: radiologic and pathologic correlation: case report. *Neurosurgery* 1996;39(5):1,031–1,034.

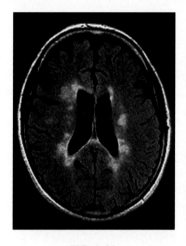

FIG. 4.1A

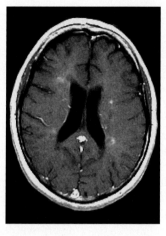

FIG. 4.1B

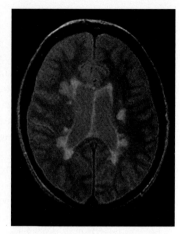

FIG. 4.1C

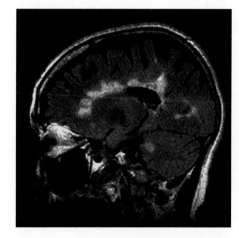

FIG. 4.1D

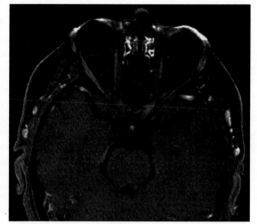

FIG. 4.1E

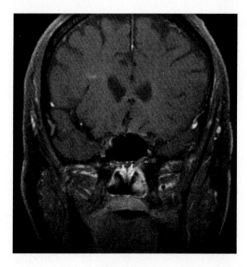

FIG. 4.1F

CLINICAL HISTORY

A 42-year-old woman with fluctuating neurological deficits over the past 10 years.

FINDINGS

Proton density, T2-weighted, and fluid-attenuated inversion-recovery (FLAIR) images demonstrate multiple periventricular abnormalities, some of which enhance following administration of gadolinium (Fig. 4.1A–D). Enhancement is also noted involving the left optic nerve (Fig. 4.1E and F). *Submitted by William G. Bradley, M.D., Ph.D., F.A.C.R., Senior Editor, Long Beach Memorial Medical Center, Long Beach, California.*

DIAGNOSIS

Multiple sclerosis (MS) and left optic neuritis.

DISCUSSION

Plaques of MS are classically ovoid in configuration with the long axis pointing perpendicular to the ependymal surface. This reflects the fact that MS is a perivenular disease and the subependymal veins course perpendicular to the ependyma. The most sensitive technique to detect demyelinating disease is thin-slice sagittal FLAIR, which demonstrates "subcallosal striations," i.e., linear lesions measuring approximately 1 mm in thickness and 2 to 3 mm in length pointing perpendicular to the ependyma (Fig. 4.1D). These lesions undoubtedly represent an early form of the classic ovoid plaque; however, they are too small to be seen on the conventional 5-mm slices used for conventional MRI of the brain. The use of 2-mm sections minimizes partial volume artifacts, while the FLAIR technique maximizes "contrast to noise." The sagittal plane is chosen to both optimally detect the undersurface of the corpus callosum and maximize the amount of white matter covered. (Because the distance from right to left is less than the distance from front to back or top to bottom, the thickness of the interslice gap can be minimized in a sagittal acquisition.)

We have not found enhanced images to increase the sensitivity of MRI for the detection of MS over and above that achievable by thin-slice sagittal FLAIR images. Nonetheless, gadolinium can be useful in discriminating a monophasic demyelinating process such as acute disseminated encephalomyelitis from a multiphasic process such as MS. Specifically, at the time of the initial diagnosis, if some of the plaques enhance and some do not, this is more suggestive of a multiphasic process such as MS than if all or none of the plaques enhance. Enhancement also has a major role in the monitoring of patients on the new immunotherapies for MS. Because T2-weighted MRI cannot readily distinguish acute from chronic MS plaques, the presence of enhancement is necessary to determine whether the immunotherapy is working. In this setting, we typically perform interleaved contiguous 3-mm T1-weighted images.

SUGGESTED READING

Palmer S, Bradley WG, Chen D-Y, et al. Subcallosal striations: early findings of multiple sclerosis on sagittal, thin-section, fast FLAIR MR images. *Radiology* 1999;210:149–153.

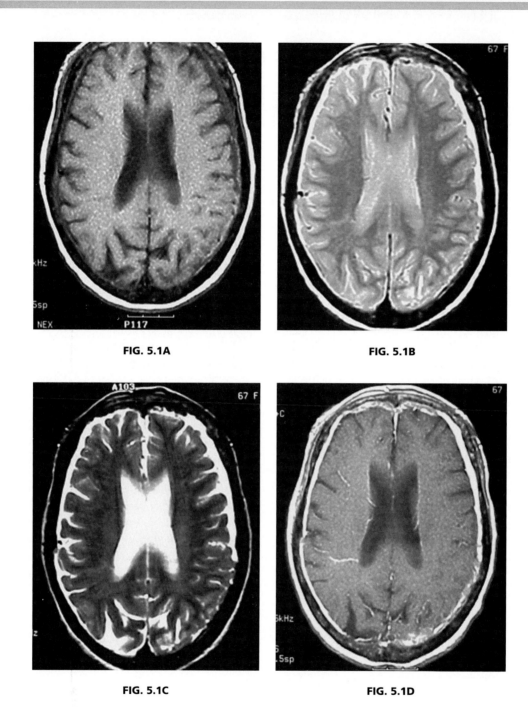

FIG. 5.1A

FIG. 5.1B

FIG. 5.1C

FIG. 5.1D

CLINICAL HISTORY

A 67-year-old woman with headache.

FINDINGS

Axial T1-weighted image (Fig. 5.1A) shows an intermediate signal rind of thickened, nodular dura over both cerebral hemispheres. The dura is thickened and hyperintense on the proton density and T2-weighted acquisition (Fig. 5.1B and C). The ventricles and sulci are normal for the patient's age. There is no parenchymal abnormality. Following contrast (Fig. 5.1D), there is intense enhancement of the dura on the T1-weighted image. Note that the abnormality does not extend into the sulci, which is indicative of dural as opposed to meningeal enhancement.

DIAGNOSIS

Metastatic dural spread of breast carcinoma.

DISCUSSION

Although the dura is quite reactive to any insult and can demonstrate thickening and enhancement in a variety of conditions, the presence of asymmetric and, particularly nodular dural disease is most often associated with metastatic spread. This typically occurs with breast carcinoma from invasion of the dura by adjacent calvarial disease. Hematogenous spread can also produce the picture in this type and other types of primary carcinoma. Differential diagnosis of asymmetric dural thickening includes sarcoidosis and infectious, as well as noninfectious causes of pachymeningitis, including idiopathic granulomatous meningitis. Primary meningioma involvement can be indistinguishable in the condition known as "diffuse meningiomatosis." Rarely, Hodgkin disease can involve the dura in an asymmetric fashion. Organized subdural or epidural hematoma from remote trauma may occasionally simulate dural metastasis.

SUGGESTED READING

Tyrell RL, Bundschun CV, Modic MT. Dural carcinomatosis: MR demonstration. *JCAT* 1987;11:329–332.
Watanabe M, Tanaka R, Takeda N. Correlation of MRI and clinical features in meningeal carcinomatosis. *Neuroradiology* 1993;35(7):512–515.

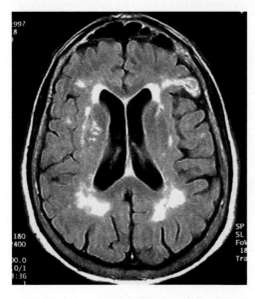

FIG. 6.1A

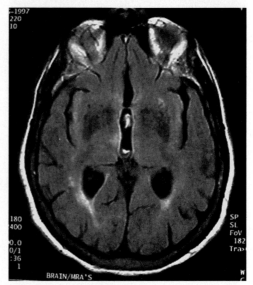

FIG. 6.1B

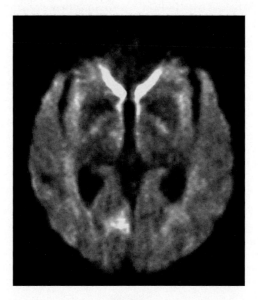

FIG. 6.1C

CLINICAL HISTORY

A 78-year-old woman with sudden loss of vision on the left.

FINDINGS

Axial fluid-attenuated inversion-recovery (FLAIR) acquisition (Fig. 6.1A and B) demonstrates multifocal deep white matter ischemic changes with a small cortical infarction in the left frontal lobe. Note no focal signal abnormality within the occipital cortex. Diffusion-weighted imaging (Fig. 6.1C) shows no abnormal high signal within the regions of infarct identified on the FLAIR image, verifying remote ischemic events. There is, however, a focus of abnormal high signal on the diffusion-weighted image within the medial right occipital lobe cortex consistent with acute infarct.

DIAGNOSIS

Acute right occipital infarct, identified only on the diffusion-weighted acquisition.

DISCUSSION

This case demonstrates the superior sensitivity of diffusion-weighted imaging when compared to conventional T2-weighted imaging and even FLAIR imaging in the detection of acute ischemic insults. The diffusion image verifies the clinical history of acute visual cortex insult. The restricted diffusion of water molecules driven into the cells in the early stages of ischemia (intracellular edema) is responsible for the signal elevation.

Subacute or chronic ischemic insults produce zones of extracellular increase in water content beginning 12 to 24 hours after the original insult, with no restriction of diffusion for water molecules therein. Diffusion restriction of acute ischemia is seen as abnormal signal on images using all three gradient directions (only one direction being shown in the figures).

Occasionally, "T2 shine through" can be seen on one or two of the gradient-selective images, and thus calculation of the diffusion coefficient may be necessary to verify the abnormal signal is representative of restricted diffusion. This is rarely necessary in the clinical setting, however. Other causes of false-positive diffusion imaging include highly proteinaceous zones of edema (e.g., in abscess cavities) and highly cellular tumors with numerous cell membranes restricting the extracellular space (e.g., melanoma metastases or very malignant metastases of any small-cell variety).

SUGGESTED READING

Baron JC, von Kummer R, Del Zoppo GJ. Treatment of acute ischemic stroke: challenging the concept of a rigid and universal time window. *Stroke* 1995;26:2,219–2,221.

Russell EJ. Diagnosis of hyperacute ischemic infarct with CT: key to improved clinical outcome after intravenous thrombolysis? *Radiology* 1997;205:315–318.

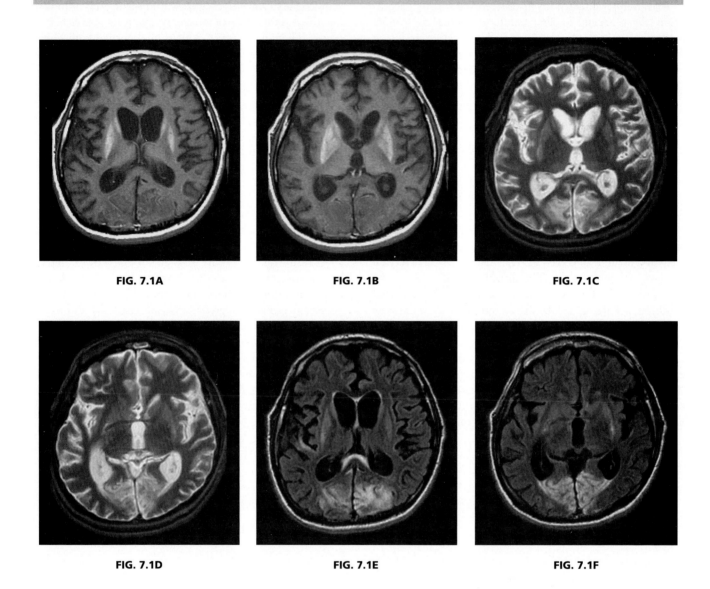

FIG. 7.1A FIG. 7.1B FIG. 7.1C

FIG. 7.1D FIG. 7.1E FIG. 7.1F

CLINICAL HISTORY

A 24-year-old man with history of motor vehicle accident and cardiopulmonary arrest 6 months earlier.

FINDINGS

There is diffuse cerebral atrophy with symmetric abnormal hyperintense signal within the lenticular nuclei and caudate heads bilaterally on T1-weighted (Fig. 7.1A and B), T2-weighted (Fig. 7.1C and D), and fluid-attenuated inversion-recovery (FLAIR) (Fig. 7.1E and F) images. Additionally, there is encephalomalacia in the occipital lobes bilaterally. *Submitted by Elizabeth Vogler, M.D., and William G. Bradley, M.D., Ph.D., F.A.C.R., Senior Editor, Long Beach Memorial Medical Center, Long Beach, California.*

DIAGNOSIS

Anoxic-ischemic insult.

DISCUSSION

Anoxic-ischemic events result in global perfusion or oxygenation disturbances rather than the usual focal ischemic events, which result in a cerebral infarct in a particular vascular territory (although the two may occur together, as in this case). Examples of anoxic-ischemic events include severe prolonged hypotension, profound asphyxia, cardiorespiratory arrest, near-drowning episode, attempted strangulation, and carbon monoxide inhalation.

MRI is the most sensitive modality for detecting the sequelae of an anoxic-ischemic event. Abnormal findings include the presence of focal or diffuse edema with or without infarction (which may be hemorrhagic), T1 hyperintensity within the basal ganglia, and laminar necrosis. Early imaging may show generalized cerebral edema, with relative sparing of the perirolandic cortex, or focal edema, with particular involvement of the occipital lobe. Late sequelae include diffuse atrophy, gliosis, and sometimes iron deposition in the thalami.

Arterial "border zone" infarcts are typical, most commonly in watershed areas between the anterior cerebral artery (ACA), the middle cerebral artery (MCA), and the posterior cerebral artery (PCA) territories. This is often seen in the parietooccipital region (ACA-MCA-PCA watershed) or in a parasagittal location at the convexities (ACA-MCA watershed). Another common pattern is generalized cortical (pseudolaminar) necrosis, which occurs within the deeper layers of the cortex where the blood supply is more precarious. Cortical necrosis is often hemorrhagic and may appear as high signal intensity serpentine, gyriform foci on T1-weighted images, and as areas of low signal intensity on follow-up studies with T2 weighting.

Characteristic signal changes are seen within the basal ganglia. Initially, T1-weighted images (Fig. 7.1A and B) demonstrate diffuse high signal intensity with indistinct borders ("fuzzy basal ganglia") while T2-weighted and FLAIR sequences demonstrate hyperintensity within the lentiform nuclei, beginning at the periphery and eventually involving the entire nucleus (Fig. 7.1C–F).

The findings differ considerably in older children or adults, term babies, and preterm babies. The findings in term babies are similar to those in older children and adults, although the findings within the basal ganglia demonstrate slightly different patterns. However, preterm babies who suffer anoxic-ischemic events are seen to develop germinal matrix hemorrhage, periventricular venous infarction, and periventricular leukomalacia. The differences in findings are thought to be related to the selective vulnerability of various parts of the brain at different stages of brain maturity.

Neonates typically develop nonprogressive neurological deficits, which are clinically referred to as "cerebral palsy." There are many different types of cerebral palsy with varied manifestations, including spastic types (spastic diplegia, quadriplegia, or hemiplegia) and nonspastic types (hyperkinetic and dystonic forms).

SUGGESTED READING

Dietrich RB. Pediatric anoxic-ischemic injury. In: Stark DD, Bradley WG, eds. *Magnetic resonance imaging,* 3rd ed. St. Louis: Mosby, 1999:1,449–1,465.

Osborn AG. *Diagnostic neuroradiology.* St. Louis: Mosby, 1994: 355–360.

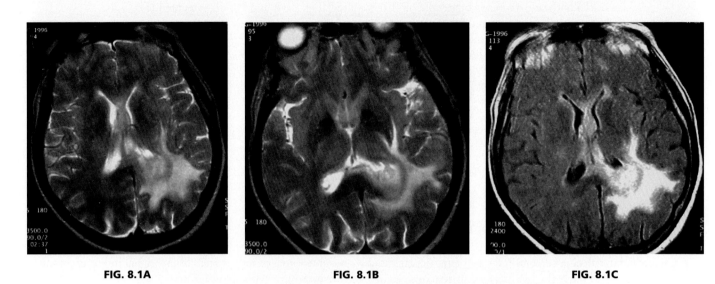

FIG. 8.1A   FIG. 8.1B   FIG. 8.1C

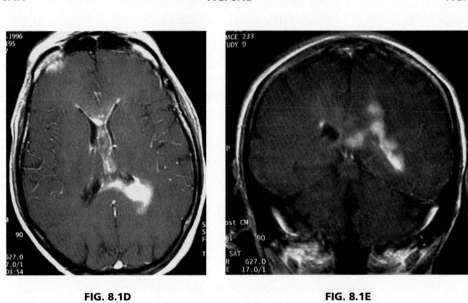

FIG. 8.1D   FIG. 8.1E

CLINICAL HISTORY

A 72-year-old woman with headache.

FINDINGS

Axial T2-weighted acquisition (Fig. 8.1A and B) demonstrates a large region of abnormal high signal involving the subcortical and deep white matter of the left parietal lobe with extension into the deep periventricular white matter. There is extension into the internal and external capsule on the left. There is minimal mass effect upon the atrium of the left lateral ventricle. Note no effacement of the overlying cortical sulci. Abnormal high signal extends across the splenium and genu of the corpus callosum (best seen on the axial fluid-attenuated inversion-recovery acquisition) (Fig. 8.1C). There is thickening and abnormal high signal at the level of the septum pellucidum. Axial and coronal postcontrast T1-weighted images (Fig. 8.1D and E) show abnormal enhancement within the deep white matter adjacent to the atrium of the left lateral ventricle extending throughout the corpus callosum and septum pellucidum. Additionally, there is enhancement along the ependymal surface of the lateral ventricles bilaterally.

DIAGNOSIS

Glioblastoma multiforme with subependymal spread of tumor.

DISCUSSION

The infiltrative nature of glioblastomas, and the fact that they represent a tumor of the brain tissue itself, results in relatively little reactive change with these tumors. Although there is vasogenic edema due to the abnormal blood–brain barrier contained within them, the hallmark of all astrocytomas (even the malignant ones) is relatively little mass effect given the size of the lesion. Other tumors (metastatic ones) would produce considerable mass effect given a similar size.

The propensity of glioblastomas to be multicentric is well known, with contiguity of the multicentric foci likely present through small avenues of infiltration on pathologic sampling. Subependymal spread and even subarachnoid seeding has been reported with malignant astrocytomas.

The abnormal vascularity of malignant astrocytomas predisposes them to in situ hemorrhage. Indeed, a small percentage (approximately 5%) of glioblastomas first present with a clinical stroke syndrome, due to acute hemorrhage into the tumor and its resultant mass effect.

SUGGESTED READING

Dean BL, Drayer BP, Bird CR, et al. Gliomas: classification with MR imaging. *Radiology* 1990;174:411–415.
Earnest IV FE, Kelly PJ, Scheithauer BW, et al. Cerebral astrocytomas: histopathologic correlation of MR and CT contrast enhancement with stereotactic biopsy. *Radiology* 1988;166:823–827.

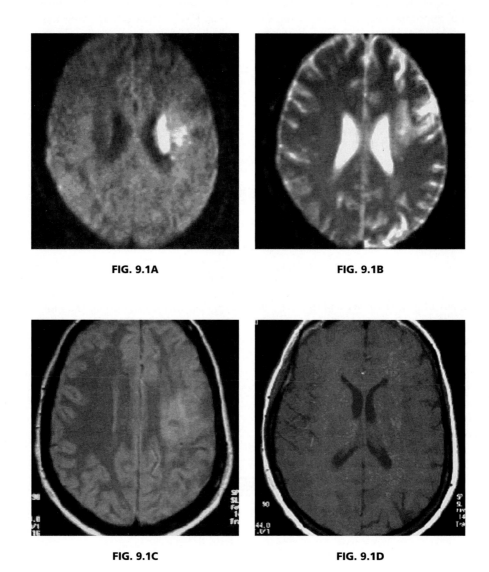

FIG. 9.1A   **FIG. 9.1B**

FIG. 9.1C   **FIG. 9.1D**

CLINICAL HISTORY

A 59-year-old man with history of atrial fibrillation and sudden onset of right hemiparesis.

FINDINGS

The diffusion image shows hyperintensity in the left corona radiata (Fig. 9.1A). On T2-weighted and proton density–weighted images, the lesion is also present but is more subtle (Fig. 9.1B and C). T1-weighted image demonstrates patchy hyperintensity in the lesion consistent with petechial hemorrhage (Fig. 9.1D). *Submitted by Sattam Lingawi, M.B., Ch.B., F.R.C.P.C., and Peter Brotchie, M.B.B.S., Ph.D., Long Beach Memorial Medical Center, Long Beach, California; William G. Bradley, M.D., Ph.D., F.A.C.R., Senior Editor.*

DIAGNOSIS

Subacute middle cerebral artery infarct.

DISCUSSION

Recently echo planar imaging (EPI) diffusion-weighted MRI has become accepted as the most effective imaging modality for the detection of acute cerebral infarctions. Several studies have shown that ischemic changes can be detected as early as 30 minutes postictus using diffusion techniques. These areas appear as strongly hyperintense foci against a relatively dark parenchymal background. In comparison, other MRI sequences (and CT) are less sensitive than diffusion-weighted imaging for detection of early ischemic injury.

T2-weighted and proton density–weighted images may show evidence of sulcal effacement and subtle increased signal intensity within the first 3 hours of onset of symptoms. Gadolinium-enhanced T1-weighted images may also show vascular stasis in the same time frame. It is primarily due to the high sensitivity and short imaging time (less than 1 minute) that EPI diffusion imaging is becoming the imaging modality of choice for evaluation of suspected infarction.

With this technique, it is important that abnormalities be present with activation of all three gradients in order to avoid misinterpreting anisotropic diffusion effects (i.e., white matter tracts oriented perpendicular to the diffusion gradient) as strokes. Alternatively, an averaged "trace" image can be used where any hyperintensity should be abnormal. If a hypertense area on the $b=1,000$ diffusion image is also hyperintense on the $b=0$ image, an apparent diffusion coefficient (ADC) map should be constructed to avoid "T2 shine through," i.e., T2 effects being the cause of high signal, not diffusion. Foci of acute ischemia appear hypointense on ADC maps while T2 shine-through remains hyperintense.

The diffusion abnormality generally represents the core infarct volume. The "ischemic penumbra," i.e., the area of brain at risk for extension of the infarct, is better estimated with the mean transit time map from the EPI perfusion study.

SUGGESTED READING

Warach S, Gaa J, Siewert B, et al. Acute human stroke studied by whole brain echo planner diffusion weighted magnetic resonance imaging. *Ann Neurol* 1995;37:231–241.

Yamada N, Imakita S, Sakuma T. Value of diffusion weighted imaging and apparent diffusion coefficient in recent cerebral infarction: a correlative study with contrast enhanced T1-weighted imaging. *AJNR* 1999;20(20):193–198.

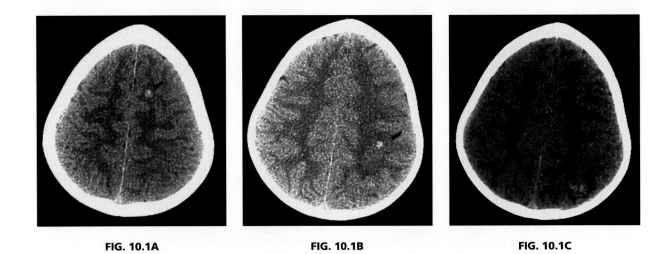

FIG. 10.1A   FIG. 10.1B   FIG. 10.1C

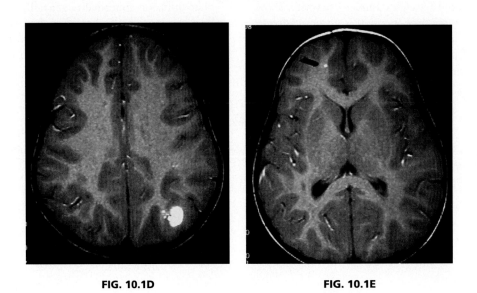

FIG. 10.1D   FIG. 10.1E

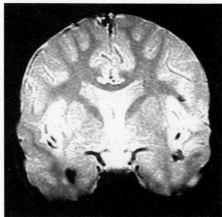
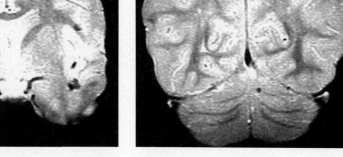

FIG. 10.1F   FIG. 10.1G

CLINICAL HISTORY

A 2-year old girl involved in a recent motor vehicle accident.

FINDINGS

Selected CT images demonstrate several subtle foci of high density at the cortical medullary junction of the left parietal lobe as well as a more diffuse, poorly defined high-density lesion at the gray-white junction of the parietooc-cipital lobe (Fig. 10.1A–C).

Axial noncontrast T1-weighted acquisition (Fig. 10.1D and E) demonstrates these lesions to be hyperintense, consistent with foci of subacute hemorrhage (methemoglobin). There is no significant perilesional edema. Coronal gradient echo acquisitions (Fig. 10.1F and G) demonstrate multiple foci of low signal consistent with deoxyhemoglobin or hemosiderin at the cortical medullary junction.

DIAGNOSIS

Shear injury.

DISCUSSION

Diffuse axonal injury (DAI) is one of the most common primary injuries to the brain in patients with severe closed head trauma. Typically, there are multiple small focal lesions scattered throughout the white matter. The injury is caused by rotationally induced shear-strain forces separating the disparately dense gray and white matter, hence the term "shear injury." Patients usually present with sudden loss of consciousness at the moment of impact. Various studies have shown that the extent of axonal injury at autopsy always exceeds that visualized on current imaging techniques, including MRI.

There are three typical regions of involvement in shear injury: the lobar white matter, the corpus callosum, and the dorsolateral aspect of the upper brainstem. The basal ganglia, thalamus, and cerebellum can also be involved. With mild head trauma, the lesions tend to occur in the lobar white matter of the frontal and temporal lobes, usually at the gray-white matter junction (stage 1). With greater severity of head trauma, the lesions will involve the posterior half of the corpus callosum (stage 2) and finally the dorsolateral aspect of the midbrain and upper pons (stage 3). Most DAI lesions are found in the lobar white matter, most commonly involving the parasagittal frontal regions and periventricular region of the temporal lobes. Occasionally, large lesions can involve the overlying cortex. Rarely, the internal and external capsule will harbor lesions.

Brainstem DAI lesions are classically located in the dorsolateral aspect of the midbrain and upper pons. There is strong predilection for certain fiber tracts including the superior cerebellar peduncles and medial lemnisci.

Occasionally, the lateral aspect of the midbrain and cerebral peduncles are involved. Lobar white matter and corpus callosum DAI lesions are virtually always present when brainstem lesions are present. If no lesions are seen in the white matter or corpus callosum, the diagnosis of brainstem axonal injury should be made with caution. The diagnosis of brainstem shear injury should not be made in the presence of transtentorial herniation or posterior fossa mass effect, both of which can produce secondary brainstem injury.

DAI lesions tend to be multiple, ovoid, or elliptical with their long axis parallel to the direction of the axonal tracts involved. Lesions range in size from 5 to 15 mm and typically show a mixture of edema and hemorrhage. Initial CT scans are often normal. Delayed imaging may, however, demonstrate findings not seen on the initial study. CT scans feature multiple tiny petechial hemorrhages at the gray-white junction and within the corpus callosum. Hemorrhagic lesions are hyperintense on T1-weighted images. The more common nonhemorrhagic lesions are difficult to identify on T1-weighted scans but present as multiple hyperintense lesions on proton density–weighted, T2-weighted, and fluid-attenuated inversion-recovery images. Hypointense lesions are seen for years after the traumatic event on T2-weighted images due to hemosiderin deposition. Gradient echo acquisition will increase the conspicuity of old hemorrhagic lesions. Nonspecific atrophic change is often a late finding in DAI.

Proton magnetic resonance spectroscopy may be a useful tool in identifying patients with DAI following closed head trauma. In a recent study, even patients with mild axonal injury demonstrated decreased N-acetylaspartate/creatine ratios in the splenium of the corpus callosum and lobar white matter.

SUGGESTED READING

Cecil KM, Hills EC, Sandel ME. Proton magnetic resonance spectroscopy for detection of axonal injury in the splenium of the corpus callosum of the brain injured patient. *J Neursurg* 1998;88(5):795–801.

Gentry LR, Thompson B, Godersley JC. MR imaging of head trauma: review of the distribution and radiopathologic features of traumatic lesions. *AJR* 1988;150(3):663–672.

Osborn AG. Craniocerebral trauma. In: *Diagnostic neuroradiology,* 1st ed. St. Louis: Mosby, 1994:213–214.

Parizel PM, Ozsarlak O, van Goethem JW, et al. MR findings in diffuse axonal injury after closed head injury. *Eur Radiol* 1998;8(6):960–965.

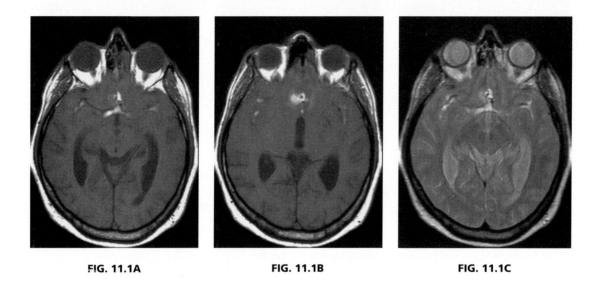

FIG. 11.1A   FIG. 11.1B   FIG. 11.1C

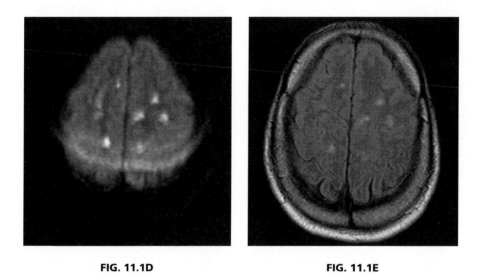

FIG. 11.1D   FIG. 11.1E

CLINICAL HISTORY

A 49-year-old man presented with marked confusion after a fall while skiing the previous week.

FINDINGS

There is diffuse subarachnoid hemorrhage with more concentrated late subacute hemorrhage in the interhemispheric fissure surrounding the anterior communicating artery (Fig. 11.1A–E). *Submitted by Elizabeth Vogler, M.D., and William G. Bradley, M.D., Ph.D., F.A.C.R., Senior Editor, Long Beach Memorial Medical Center, Long Beach, California.*

DIAGNOSIS

Subarachnoid hemorrhage due to ruptured anterior communicating artery aneurysm.

DISCUSSION

Aneurysm rupture is the most common cause of non-traumatic subarachnoid hemorrhage. Berry aneurysms are the most common type of intracranial aneurysm. They typically occur at the bifurcations of major arteries, and 80% to 90% involve the internal carotid bifurcation, anterior and posterior communicating arteries, and the bifurcation of the middle cerebral arteries.

Patients present with severe headache, nuchal rigidity, and altered level of consciousness. Besides causing subarachnoid hemorrhage, a ruptured aneurysm can also result in intraparenchymal, subdural, and intraventricular hemorrhage. The location is often a clue in determining the site of bleeding. For example, blood in the sylvian fissure is usually related to a ruptured aneurysm from the ipsilateral internal carotid, middle cerebral, or posterior communicating artery, whereas blood in the interhemispheric fissure is usually related to an aneurysm of the anterior communicating artery. Subarachnoid blood should clear from the cerebrospinal fluid (CSF) within 1 week.

Vasospasm can occur 72 to 96 hours after the initial hemorrhage and lead to ischemic infarcts, thus increasing morbidity significantly. Additionally, rebleeding of the aneurysm occurs in 20% of ruptured aneurysms within 2 weeks of the initial event and carries a 3% risk of rebleeding in patients surviving 6 months after the initial bleed. Overall, mortality is approximately 60%. Another complication of subarachnoid hemorrhage is communicating hydrocephalus, caused by blockage of the arachnoid villa resulting in impaired resorption of CSF. This may require shunting.

CT is most commonly used for diagnosis of subarachnoid hemorrhage. However, recent studies have shown fluid-attenuated inversion-recovery (FLAIR) sequences to be 100% sensitive in detecting acute subarachnoid hemorrhage. Subarachnoid and intraventricular hemorrhage differ from intraparenchymal hemorrhage because they are mixed with CSF and have higher oxygen tension. Immediately upon mixing CSF with subarachnoid hemorrhage, the protein content is increased and the T1 is shortened. Therefore, bloody CSF appears hyperintense of FLAIR sequences (where it is normally nulled and should appear black). Late subacute hemorrhage also appears bright on diffusion imaging (Fig. 11.1D) due to restricted water motion.

SUGGESTED READING

Bradley WG. Hemorrhage. In: Stark DD, Bradley WG, eds. *Magnetic resonance imaging,* 3rd ed. St. Louis: Mosby, 1999;1,329–1,346.

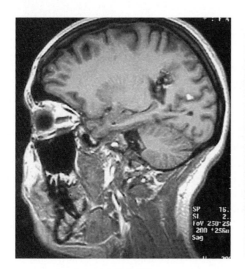

FIG. 12.1A

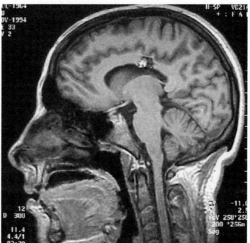

FIG. 12.1B

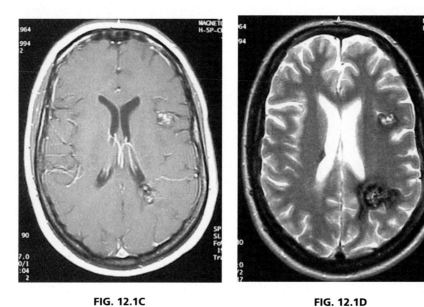

FIG. 12.1C   **FIG. 12.1D**

CLINICAL HISTORY

A 30-year-old woman with new seizure.

FINDINGS

Parasagittal T1-weighted images (Fig. 12.1A and B) demonstrate multiple subcortical and deep periventricular lesions. These lesions are characterized by central hyperintensity with a well-circumscribed border of low signal (a popcorn appearance). Axial postcontrast T1-weighted image (Fig. 12.1C) demonstrates no significant enhancement of these lesions. Axial T2-weighted images (Fig. 12.1D) shows the typical popcornlike lesions with central regions of hyperintensity and hypointense peripheral rims consistent with multiple foci of subacute hemorrhage with hemosiderin at the periphery. There are no abnormal feeding arteries or draining veins identified.

DIAGNOSIS

Multifocal cavernous angiomas.

DISCUSSION

Intracranial vascular malformations are traditionally divided into four categories: arteriovenous malformation, the capillary telangiectasia, the venous angioma (developmental venous anomaly), and the cavernous angioma (cavernous hemangioma, cavernoma, or cavernous malformation). These are four distinct histologic entities; however, they can overlap each other. Different types of vascular malformations can occur in the same patient. The most common association is between the cavernous angioma and venous angioma, reported to occur in 8% to 33% of cases (see Volume 2, Case 67).

Cavernous angiomas account for 8% to 16% of all cerebral vascular malformations. They are typically angiographically occult, hence, the commonly used term "occult cerebrovascular malformation." Pathologically, they are endothelial-lined sinusoidal vascular spaces without intervening normal neural tissue that contain blood in various stages of degradation. Typically, there is a peripheral rim of hemosiderin deposition. They are thought to be congenital but usually are first discovered in the third to fifth decade of life. The lesions are usually asymptomatic but can produce focal neurological deficits following hemorrhage. Seizure is a common presenting complaint. Hemorrhages are usually small and of low pressure, resulting in slow expansion of these lesions. Recurrent occult hemorrhage is common. It is rarely life threatening. Cavernomas can occur in the brain or spinal cord. They tend to be superficial or subcortical when in the brain, usually in close proximity to the subarachnoid space or ventricles. Ten percent occur deep within the basal ganglia, thalami, or internal capsules. Approximately 25% are infratentorial, involving the brainstem or cerebellum.

The pons is the most common infratentorial site. Rarely the leptomeninges or cranial nerves are involved. Cavernous angiomas can be multiple (50%) and in such cases tend to be familial.

On CT, cavernous angiomas are isodense to hyperdense lesions on noncontrast images and are often associated with calcification and gliosis. Enhancement results are variable. The classic MRI appearance is described as "popcornlike." There is a central reticulated core of heterogeneous signal on all pulse sequences due to blood in various stages of evolution. Most commonly, the blood is in the subacute stage (methemoglobin) and is hyperintense on T1-weighted and T2-weighted images. A complete smooth rim of low signal surrounds cavernous angiomas on all pulse sequences due to the peripheral hemosiderin deposition. Gradient echo imaging detects these lesions with greater sensitivity due to the susceptibility effects of hemosiderin. Gradient echo imaging sequences make the low signal hemosiderin within the cavernoma "bloom," increasing lesion conspicuity. In a significant number of cases, multiple cavernomas are shown with gradient echo imaging, whereas none or only one is seen on conventional sequences.

Cavernous angiomas can be difficult to differentiate from other hemorrhagic lesions such as metastases. The presence of a relatively smooth, complete hypointense rim of hemosiderin is an important observation in the diagnosis of cavernoma, as is the lack of surrounding edema and mass effect. Hemorrhagic tumor more typically has an irregular incomplete rim of low signal. Primary hemorrhage without underlying pathologic focus should resolve within 4 to 6 weeks.

SUGGESTED READING

Barker CS. MRI of intracranial cavernous angiomas: a report of 13 cases with pathologic confirmation. *Clin Radiol* 1993;48(2):117–121.

Osborn AG. Intracranial vascular malformations. In: *Diagnostic neuroradiology*, 1st ed. St. Louis: Mosby, 1994:311–313.

Rabinov JD. Diagnostic imaging of angiographically occult vascular malformations. *Neurosurg Clin North Am* 1999;10(3):419–432.

Tomlinson FH, Houser OW, Scheithauer BW, et al. Angiographically occult vascular malformations: a correlative study of features on MRI and histologic examination. *Neurosurgery* 1994;34(5):792–799.

Wagner BJ, Richardson KJ, Moran AM, et al. Intracranial vascular malformations. *Semin Ultrasound Comput Tomogr Magn Reson* 1995;16(3):253–268.

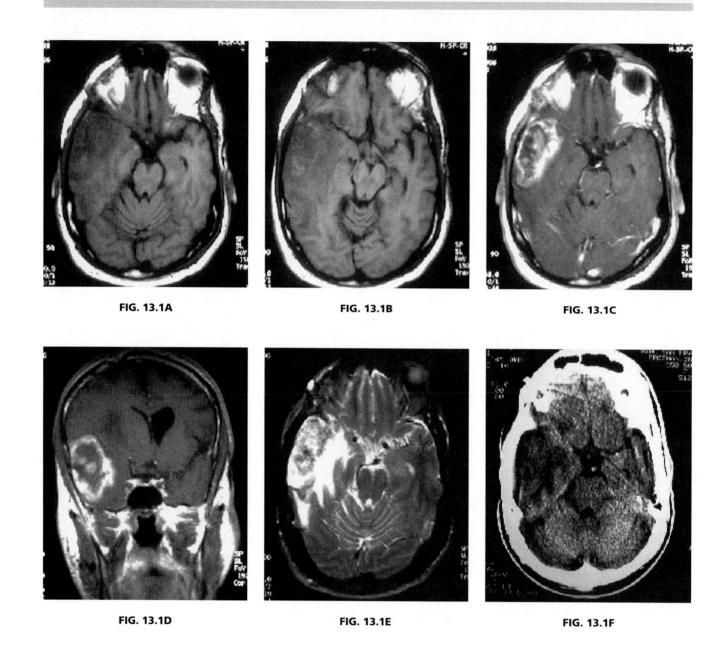

FIG. 13.1A   **FIG. 13.1B**   **FIG. 13.1C**

FIG. 13.1D   **FIG. 13.1E**   **FIG. 13.1F**

CLINICAL HISTORY

A 63-year-old man 18 months after whole brain radiation for glioblastoma multiforme.

FINDINGS

T1-weighted images show a large mass in the right temporal lobe with areas of necrosis (Fig. 13.1A and B) and ring enhancement (Fig. 13.1C and D). T2-weighted image shows surrounding edema (Fig. 13.1E) more prominently than CT (Fig. 13.1F). *Submitted by Kathleen Flores, M.D., Peter Brotchie, M.B.B.S., Ph.D., Sattam Lingawi, M.B., Ch.B., F.R.C.P.C., and William G. Bradley, M.D., Ph.D., F.A.C.R., Senior Editor, Long Beach Memorial Medical Center, Long Beach, California.*

DIAGNOSIS

Radiation necrosis.

DISCUSSION

On conventional magnetic resonance images, radiation necrosis cannot be distinguished from recurrent glioblastoma. Using magnetic resonance spectroscopy, radiation necrosis has a low choline peak while glioblastoma multiforme has high choline. (Radiation-induced white matter change also has elevated choline.)

There are seven main forms of radiation-induced damage to the central nervous system (CNS):

1. Focal CNS necrosis occurs preferentially at the tumor site and appears as a ring-enhancing lesion with surrounding edema and mass effect. The patient is usually clinically deteriorating and has increased intracranial pressure. Magnetic resonance spectroscopy can be useful in differentiating this entity from tumor recurrence by demonstrating a large lipid peak and minimal choline, although the two entities may occur together (particularly following radiosurgery or brachytherapy).

2. Diffuse white matter injury is seen in up to 40% of postradiation cases and results in periventricular, deep white matter demyelination and elevated carbon dioxide level. The MRI appearance is similar to that of deep white matter ischemia. Diffuse necrotizing leukoencephalomyelopathy is a subcategory with similar MRI appearance to that seen as a result of combined radiation therapy and intrathecal chemotherapy.

3. CNS atrophy involves the cerebral hemispheres and the cerebellum.

4. Mineralizing microangiopathy is due to dystrophic calcification of hyalinized and obliterated small vessels, and most often occurs in the basal ganglia in children.

5. Large vessel vasculopathy involves intracranial and extracranial vessels and results in vessel occlusion secondary to intimal proliferation and accelerated atherosclerosis.

6. Optic neuropathy occurs as a result of sellar and parasellar radiation. Initially, the optic nerves are swollen and enhance with gadolinium. However, they eventually atrophy with probable loss of vision.

7. Telangiectasia is believed to be due to dilation of small vessels and capillaries as a response to venous thrombosis and radiation-induced vascular occlusion. This may result in foci of subclinical hemorrhage.

SUGGESTED READING

Rabin BM, Meyer JR, Berlin JW, et al. Radiation-induced changes in the central nervous system and head and neck. *Radiographics* 1996;16:1,055–1,072.

Tsuruda JS, Kortman KE, Bradley WG, et al. Radiation effects on cerebral white matter: MR evaluation. *AJR* 1987;149(1):165–171.

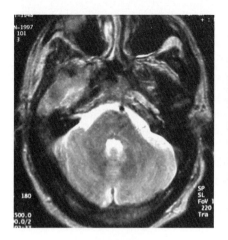

FIG. 14.1A

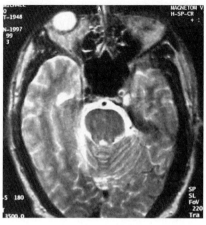

FIG. 14.1B

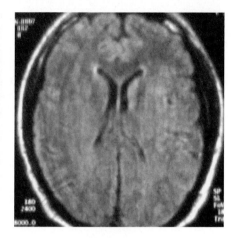

FIG. 14.1C

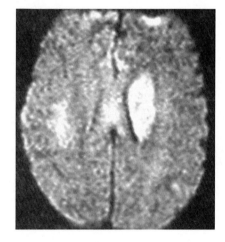

FIG. 14.1D

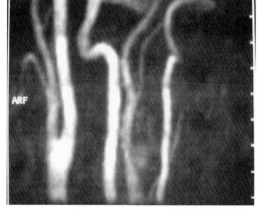

FIG. 14.1E

CLINICAL HISTORY

A 49-year-old man with acute onset of right-sided weakness.

FINDINGS

Axial T2-weighted image (Fig. 14.1A) demonstrates lack of normal flow void within the internal carotid artery on the left at the skull base. More superiorly (Fig. 14.1B), within the cavernous portion of the left internal carotid artery, there is a peripheral crescentic collection of high signal on the T2-weighted acquisition, consistent with intramural thrombus. Compare this to the normal right internal carotid artery where there is normal flow void. The axial fluid-attenuated inversion-recovery image (Fig. 14.1C) demonstrates no signal abnormality within the brain. The diffusion-weighted images (Fig. 14.1D) show an abnormal focus of high signal in the left basal ganglia, consistent with acute infarction. Magnetic resonance angiogram (MRA) (Fig. 14.1E) shows a normal distal right common carotid artery, as well as normal right internal and external carotid arteries. There is marked narrowing of the cervical left internal carotid artery.

DIAGNOSIS

Acute left internal carotid artery dissection with acute basal ganglia infarct seen only on the diffusion-weighted image.

DISCUSSION

Carotid artery dissection is typically classified as traumatic or spontaneous (atraumatic). Spontaneous carotid artery dissection is now one of the most frequent causes of ischemic stroke in young patients. It accounts for 2% of all strokes but 20% of ischemic strokes that occur in patients who are less than 45 years of age. Spontaneous dissection is commonly associated with one of several disease states wherein there is an intrinsic abnormality of the vessel wall, including fibromuscular dysplasia, Marfan syndrome, Ehlers-Danlos syndrome, and cystic medial necrosis. Spontaneous craniocervical artery dissection can also result from physical exertion, strenuous exercise, and even minor seemingly negligible trauma. Any cause of acute hypertension can result in carotid artery dissection.

A dissection occurs when blood penetrates the intima and extends a variable distance within the vessel wall (usually in a cephalad direction). The dissection is typically subintimal, resulting in narrowing of the involved vessel lumen. The reduced flow within the involved vessel promotes thrombus formation, leading to embolic complications and vessel occlusion. Pseudoaneurysm formation is an uncommon complication resulting from subadventitial dissection of blood.

Patients with internal carotid artery dissection most often present with headaches, typically described as "orbital" or "periorbital" in location. Neck pain, signs of cerebral ischemia, and Horner syndrome are common presenting complaints.

Carotid dissection most often afflicts the cervical internal carotid artery, rarely extending beyond the skull base. It usually spares the carotid bulb, beginning approximately 2 cm distal to the carotid bifurcation. Multivessel involvement is reported in one third of cases.

MRI and three-dimensional (3D) time-of-flight (TOF) MR angiography are both used as reliable, noninvasive methods of assessing internal carotid artery dissection. The sensitivity and specificity of both MRI and MRA in the diagnosis of carotid artery dissection has been reported to be 84% to 99%. The percentages are lower for vertebral artery dissection.

The advantages of MRI and MRA over conventional angiography include the ability to view an infinite number of projections of the artery, to actually visualize the intramural hematoma, and to assess the intracranial circulation and evaluate for associated cerebral infarction.

Criteria for diagnosis of dissection on MRI and MRA include direct visualization of the hematoma within the vessel wall, an increased external diameter of the involved artery and narrowing of the vessel lumen. On MRI, the mural hematoma appears as a crescentic collection of abnormal signal along the vessel wall adjacent to signal void within the residual patent vessel lumen. The signal intensity within the hematoma depends on its age. In the subacute stage, which is most commonly seen, the signal is hyperintense on T1-weighted and T2-weighted images because of the paramagnetic effects of methemoglobin. If the hematoma is acute (1 to 4 days), the signal is low on both T1-weighted and T2-weighted images, making the diagnosis more difficult. It is the intramural hematoma that widens the external diameter of the involved vessel on MRA—a finding that has been shown to be the most reliable indicator of internal carotid artery dissection. An intimal flap is rarely seen on MRI or MRA.

Caution should be taken when evaluating 3D TOF maximum intensity projection (MIP) images, as differentiation between normal hyperintense flow within the vessel and high signal intramural thrombus can be difficult. The source images from the MRA should always be consulted. Fat-saturated T1-weighted MRI is helpful in identifying intramural hematoma.

The intramural hematoma seen in internal carotid artery dissection is nicely demonstrated in this case on T2-weighted acquisition. There is narrowing of the vessel lumen on 3D TOF MRA MIP images.

SUGGESTED READING

Bui LN, Brant-Zawadzki MN, Vergbese P, et al. Magnetic resonance angiography of cervicocranial dissection. *Stroke* 1993;24:126–131.

Klufas RA, Hsu L, Barnes PD, et al. Dissection of the carotid and vertebral arteries: imaging with magnetic resonance angiography. *AJR* 1995;164(3):673–677.

Levy C, Laissy JP, Raveau V, et al. Carotid and vertebral artery dissection: 3D time of flight magnetic resonance angiography and MR imaging versus conventional angiography. *Radiology* 1994;190(1):97–103.

Oelerich M, Stogbaurer F, Kurlemann G, et al. Craniocervical artery dissection: MR imaging and MR angiography findings. *Eur Radiol* 1999;9(7):1,385–1,391.

Ozdoba C, Surzenegger M, Schroth G. Internal carotid artery dissection: MR imaging features and clinical and radiologic correlation. *Radiology* 1996;199(1):191–198.

Provenzale JM, Barboriak DP, Taveras JM. Exercise-related dissection of craniocervical arteries: CT, MR, and angiography findings. *JCAT* 1995;19(2):268–276.

Russo CP, Smoker WRK. Nonatheromatous carotid artery disease. *Neuroimaging Clin North Am* 1996;6(4):811–830.

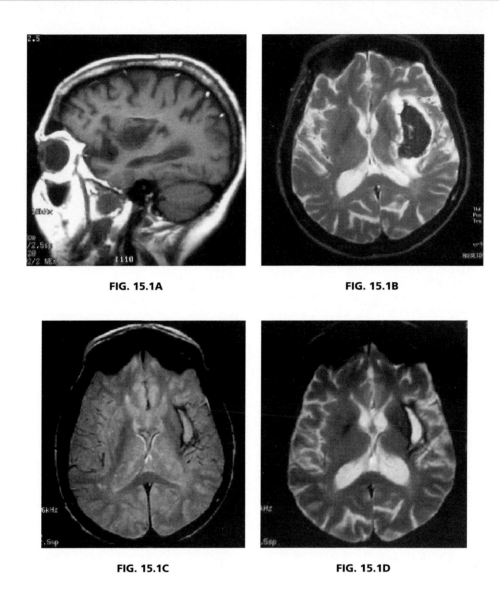

FIG. 15.1A

FIG. 15.1B

FIG. 15.1C

FIG. 15.1D

CLINICAL HISTORY

A 63-year-old woman with history of hypertension and a sudden onset of right hemiparesis.

FINDINGS

There is a low-intensity mass in the left basal ganglia on the T1-weighted image, which turns very dark on the T2-weighted image (Fig. 15.1A and B). *Submitted by Peter Brotchie, M.B.B.S., Ph.D., Sattam Lingawi, M.B., Ch.B., F.R.C.P.C., and William G. Bradley, M.D., Ph.D., F.A.C.R., Senior Editor, Long Beach Memorial Medical Center, Long Beach, California.*

DIAGNOSIS

Acute hypertensive hemorrhage.

DISCUSSION

The low-intensity mass is consistent with intracellular deoxyhemoglobin from acute hemorrhage. A small focus of hyperintensity is seen within the mass on the T2-weighted image, consistent with oxyhemoglobin. Mild vasogenic edema surrounds the hemorrhage, which is situated predominantly within the external capsule, extending into the putamen (Fig. 15.1B). These images were obtained a day after the onset of symptoms. Figures 15.1C and D were obtained 4 weeks later, demonstrating increased signal centrally within the hematoma on the proton density–weighted and T2-weighted images, consistent with extracellular methemoglobin, surrounded by a low-intensity rim of hemosiderin (chronic hemorrhage).

The different paramagnetic forms of hemoglobin and the intracellular versus extracellular environment lead to a characteristic MRI appearance of evolving parenchymal hemorrhage. Hyperacute hemorrhage (first few hours) contains oxyhemoglobin, acute hemorrhage (days 1 to 3) contains deoxyhemoglobin, subacute hemorrhage (up to 3 weeks) contains methemoglobin, and chronic hemorrhage (more than 2 months) has a hemosiderin rim. Subacute hemorrhage can be further divided into "early" and "late" forms, depending on the time of red cell lysis. Early subacute hemorrhage (intracellular methemoglobin) appears after approximately 3 days and lasts for about a week. The late subacute phase (extracellular methemoglobin) appears after approximately 1 week. The chronic phase is defined on MRI by the presence of a hemosiderin rim surrounding the free methemoglobin and hemichromes (nonparamagnetic proteinaceous heme derivatives) (Table 15.1).

TABLE 15.1

Time	Composition	T1-weighted image	T2-weighted image
Hyperacute (<24 hours)	Oxyhemoglobin	Isointense	Hyperintense
Acute (1–3 days)	Deoxyhemoglobin	Hypointense	Hypointense
Early subacute (3–7 days)	Intracellular methemoglobin	Hyperintense	Hypointense
Late subacute (1–2 weeks)	Extracellular methemoglobin	Hyperintense	Hyperintense
Chronic (>2 weeks)	Hemosiderin rim	Hypointense	Hypointense

SUGGESTED READING

Bradley WG. MR appearance of hemorrhage in the brain. *Radiology* 1993;189:15–26.

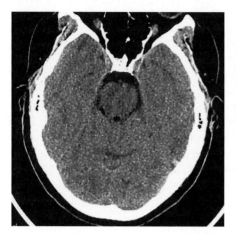

FIG. 16.1A

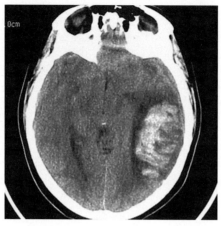

FIG. 16.1B

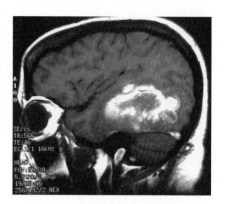

FIG. 16.1C

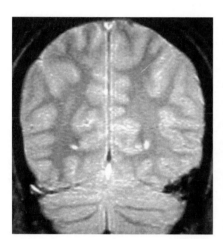

FIG. 16.1D

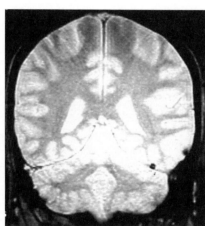

FIG. 16.1E

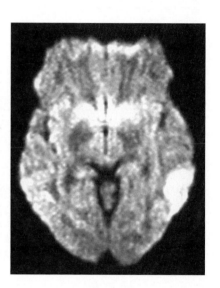

FIG. 16.1F

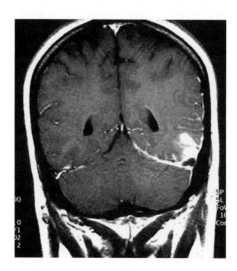

FIG. 16.1G

CLINICAL HISTORY

A 25-year-old woman with acute onset of aphasia and disorientation.

FINDINGS

The initial CT scan acquired in the emergency department (Fig. 16.1A) demonstrates very subtle low density within the cortex and subcortical white matter of the posterior temporal lobe on the left. There is a tiny focus of high density suggestive of hemorrhage. A follow-up study acquired 3 days later demonstrates marked abnormality in the left temporal lobe (Fig. 16.1B), characterized by a large region of high density consistent with acute hemorrhage with associated perifocal edema. Sagittal T1-weighted acquisition (Fig. 16.1C) confirms a large hemorrhagic lesion within the left temporal lobe. The peripheral high signal is due to methemoglobin effect. There is isointense material, centrally suggestive of acute blood. Also note the abnormal high signal within the transverse sinus consistent with very slow flow or thrombosis. Coronal gradient echo acquisition (Fig. 16.1D and E) shows loss of normal high signal flow within the left transverse sinus as well as the several cortical veins, consistent with fresh thrombus. Compare with the normal right transverse sinus. Diffusion-weighted image (Fig. 16.1F) shows abnormal high signal within the posterior left temporal lobe consistent with acute infarction. Coronal postcontrast T1-weighted image (Fig. 16.1G) shows no enhancement of the transverse sinus. There is meningeal enhancement along the left leaf of the tentorium and along the surface of the left temporal lobe as well as intravascular enhancement—all findings associated with acute infarction. The mastoid air cells are clear.

DIAGNOSIS

Acute hemorrhagic venous infarct within the posterior left temporal lobe secondary to acute thrombosis of the left transverse sinus.

DISCUSSION

This case serves to illustrate the subtle early appearance of venous infarction and its dramatic evolution over a short interval into a combination of infarction of a hemorrhage. The clinical picture is often staggered over hours or days. Venous thrombosis leads to loss of perfusion in the regional segment of the brain drained by the occluded vein while inflow to the region is maintained. The loss of perfusion pressure produces the initial ischemic insult, and the continued arterial inflow in the face of no outflow leads to the subsequent hemorrhage. Although venous infarction can be isolated, it is typically associated with thrombosis in a dural sinus as well. Institution of thrombolytic therapy in the earliest stages of dural sinus thrombosis (if recognized) can prevent the hemorrhagic evolution and minimize the ischemic insult.

With dural sinus thrombosis, intracranial pressure elevation produces headache, and papilledema may be observed. The actual infarction leads to focal neurological findings or seizure, the ensuing hemorrhage aggravating the condition.

Typical causes of venous/dural sinus thrombosis include the use of oral contraceptive pills or the peripartum/postpartum state in women, any other source of hypercoaguability, including blood dyscrasias, dehydration, paraneoplastic syndromes, certain chemotherapeutic regimens, as well as infection of adjacent bone or calvarial sinus, including sinusitis, mastoiditis, middle-ear infection, or calvarial osteomyelitis. Direct tumor invasion can lead to dural sinus occlusion but is a rare cause of acute sinus thrombosis due to the slow progression of the process, allowing collateralization of the venous pathways. The tentorial enhancement in this case is an example of collateralization through tentorial veins for the occluded sinus.

Hemorrhagic stroke may be the first presentation of venous infarction/thrombosis; such hemorrhages differ from other spontaneous bleeds (e.g., hypertension) in that they often exhibit considerable surrounding edema (from preexisting infarction) as opposed to hypertensive bleeds.

SUGGESTED READING

Alexandrov AV, Black SE, Ehrlich LE, et al. Predictors of hemorrhagic transformation occuring spontaneously and on anticoagulants in patients with acute ischemic stroke. *Stroke* 1997;28:1,198–1,202.

Larrue V, von Kummer R, del Zoppo G, et al. Hemorrhagic transformation in acute ischemic stroke. *Stroke* 1997;28:957–960.

Motto C, Ciccone A, Aritzu E, et al. Hemorrhage after an acute ischemic stroke. *Stroke* 1999;30:761–764.

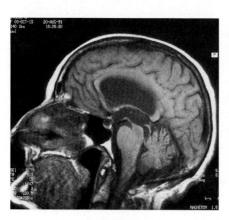

FIG. 17.1A

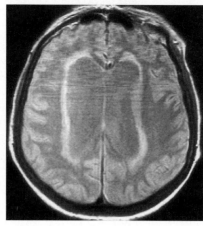

FIG. 17.1B

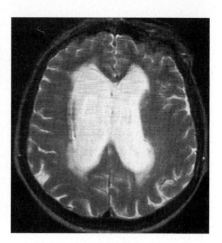

FIG. 17.1C

CLINICAL HISTORY

A 77-year-old woman with dementia and gait disturbance.

FINDINGS

The T1-weighted sagittal image demonstrates upward bowing of the corpus callosum, indicating hydrocephalus. The aqueduct is flared proximally but narrows to a point distally, suggesting stenosis (Fig. 17.1A). Proton density–weighted and T2-weighted axial sections through the lateral ventricles demonstrate hydrocephalus with sur-rounding deep white matter ischemic changes (Fig. 17.1B and C). There is no evidence of high signal under the genu or splenium of the corpus callosum to indicate interstitial edema from acute obstruction. *Submitted by William G. Bradley, M.D., Ph.D., F.A.C.R., Senior Editor, Long Beach Memorial Medical Center, Long Beach, California.*

DIAGNOSIS

Aqueductal stenosis.

DISCUSSION

While aqueductal stenosis is usually a prenatal diagnosis made by ultrasound, it can occasionally present later in life with signs of increased intracranial pressure. Typically, this presentation occurs in the late 30s or 40s and more commonly in women than in men. Although there are a number of forms of aqueductal stenosis that are not compatible with life, these late-presentation cases most likely involve an aqueductal membrane with a pinhole allowing some cerebrospinal fluid (CSF) flow. Early in life, the ventricles dilate and a metastable equilibrium is reached such that the amount of CSF produced by the choroid plexus manages to get through the pinhole in the aqueductal membrane without backing up further. Then, later in life, a slight increase in CSF production upsets this equilibrium and probably accounts for the additional ventricular enlargement and new onset of symptoms.

This patient's case is unusual in that she first sought medical attention at age 73. In view of her age, normal pressure hydrocephalus was considered the most likely diagnosis following CT; however, the sagittal view on MRI clearly demonstrates the lack of aqueductal patency. The lack of an aqueductal CSF flow void further attests to this diagnosis. The normal size of the fourth ventricle also suggests obstructive, rather than communicating, hydrocephalus, e.g., NPH.

The hyperintensity surrounding the lateral ventricles in this elderly patient is confined to the lateral aspect of the lateral ventricular walls, a site favored by small vessel ischemic change. Although there is a passing resemblance to interstitial edema, these small vessel ischemic changes are much less regular than the smooth margins produced by transependymal resorption of CSF. The latter also tends to occur around the entire ventricle, including the undersurface of the splenium and genu of the corpus callosum (which is not involved here).

SUGGESTED READING

Barkovich AJ, Newton TH. MR of aqueductal stenosis: evidence of a broad spectrum of tectal distortion. *Am J Neuroradiol* 1989;30:471.

McMillian JJ, Williams B. Aqueduct stenosis. *J Neurol Neurosurg Psychiatry* 1977;93:679.

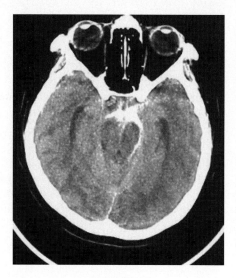

FIG. 18.1A

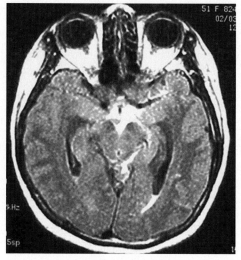

FIG. 18.1B

CLINICAL HISTORY

A 51-year-old man with acute onset of intense headache.

FINDINGS

Axial noncontrast CT (Fig. 18.1A) shows abnormal high-density material within the prepontine and ambient cisterns. Axial fluid-attenuated inversion-recovery (FLAIR) acquisition performed on the same day (Fig. 18.1B) shows high signal in the same distribution.

DIAGNOSIS

Acute subarachnoid hemorrhage.

DISCUSSION

Fluid-attenuated inversion-recovery sequences are designed to suppress all signal from hydrogen nuclei within pure spinal fluid. However, the addition of proteinaceous or hemorrhagic component to cerebrospinal fluid (CSF) produces signal intensity elevation within it on FLAIR acquisition. Thus, this has become an essential sequence for brain imaging and is the most sensitive way of detecting acute subarachnoid hemorrhage, as well as other conditions affecting CSF protein content such as infectious meningitis and carcinomatous infiltration of the meninges.

Even CT scanning can miss acute subarachnoid hemorrhage in a small number of cases; thus, a high degree of clinical suspicion in the face of negative brain scans still necessitates lumbar puncture (the gold standard) to verify or exclude the presence of subarachnoid hemorrhage or acute meningitis. Occasionally, pulsation-related phase artifact can simulate subarachnoid hemorrhage on FLAIR sequences in the prepontine space; thus, careful attention to technique and experience with one's instrument is necessary in subtle cases of prepontine subarachnoid hemorrhage. CT or lumbar puncture can be performed if confusion persists.

SUGGESTED READING

Hayman LA, Pagani JJ, Kirkpatrick JB, et al. Pathophysiology of acute intracranial and subarachnoid hemorrhage: applications to MR imaging. *AJNR* 1989;10:457–461.

Jenkins A, Hadley DM, Teasdale GM, et al. Magnetic resonance imaging of acute subarachnoid hemorrhage. *J Neurosurg* 1988;68:731–736.

Noguchi K, Ogawa T, Inugami A, et al. MR of acute subarachnoid hemorrhage: a preliminary report of fluid-attenuated inversion-recovery pulse sequences. *AJNR* 1994;15:1,940–1,943.

Tatter SB, Buonanno FS, Ogilvy CS. Acute lacunar stroke in association with angiogram-negative subarachnoid hemorrhage. *Stroke* 1995;26:891–895.

Vehlthuis BK, Rinkel GJE, Ramos LMP, et al. Perimesencephalic hemorrhage. *Stroke* 1999;30:1,103–1,109.

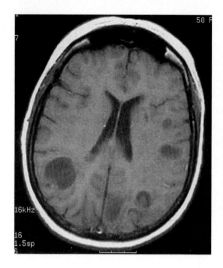

FIG. 19.1A

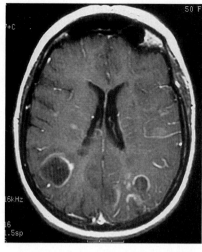

FIG. 19.1B

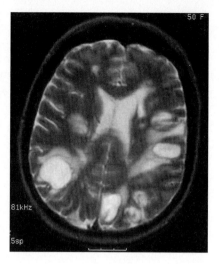

FIG. 19.1C

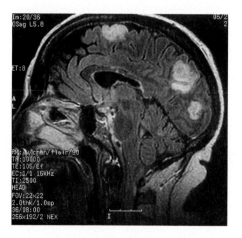

FIG. 19.1D

CLINICAL HISTORY

A 51-year-old woman with history of multiple sclerosis (MS) and new onset seizures.

FINDINGS

There are multiple incomplete ring-enhancing lesions involving the white matter of both cerebral hemispheres (Fig. 19.1A and B), which are bright on a T2-weighted image (Fig. 19.1C) and a fluid-attenuated inversion-recovery (FLAIR) image (Fig. 19.1D). *Submitted by Sangita Patel, M.D., William B. Bradley, M.D., Ph.D., F.A.C.R., Senior Editor, Long Beach Memorial Medical Center, Long Beach, California.*

DIAGNOSIS

Tumefactive MS.

DISCUSSION

MS is a chronic inflammatory demyelinating disease of unknown etiology. Peak age at presentation is 25 to 30 years with a female predominance of 2:1. Presenting symptoms include headaches, dizziness, nausea, and recurrent sensory changes, as well as weakness, ataxia, and diplopia. There are both acute and chronic stages. Lack of eye, sensory, bladder, and cerebrospinal fluid abnormalities suggest a diagnosis other than MS or as its monophasic counterpart, acute disseminated encephalomyelitis (ADEM).

MS lesions are usually subependymal or pericallosal in location. They usually do not have mass effect or edema unless they are acute. The classic "Dawson's fingers" are ovoid lesions oriented perpendicular to the ventricles. In their earliest form, they produce "subcallosal striations," i.e., fine ovoid-linear structures on the undersurface of the corpus callosum, best seen on thin-slice sagittal FLAIR images (Fig. 19.1D). They are the result of periventricular demyelination. As is seen in this case, MS may also present as mass lesions with enhancement, i.e., "tumefactive MS." It is only really distinguished from ADEM by history, although the presence of some enhancing and some nonenhancing lesions on MRI suggests a multiphasic process such as that of MS. The age of the patient and sparing of the gray matter can help in making the diagnosis and excluding other diagnoses such as tumor and other inflammatory processes.

MRI shows discrete foci of varying size with high signal on proton density T2-weighted and FLAIR images and corresponding hypointense signal on T1-weighted images. A "fried egg" appearance is typical (Fig. 19.1C) (i.e., brighter plaque [yolk] surrounded by less bright edema [bright]). Partial rim enhancement can be seen up to 8 weeks following an acute episode.

SUGGESTED READING

Lakhanpal SK, Maravilla KR. Multiple sclerosis. In: Stark DD, Bradley WG, eds. *Magnetic resonance imaging,* 3rd ed. St. Louis: Mosby, 1999:1,379–1,402.

Palmer S, Bradley WG, Chen D-Y, et al. Subcallosal striations: early findings of multiple sclerosis on sagittal, thin-section, fast FLAIR MR images. *Radiology* 1999;210:149–153.

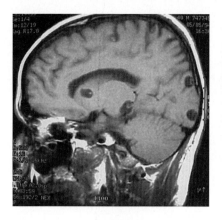

FIG. 20.1A

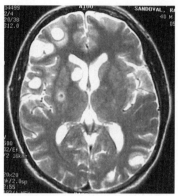

FIG. 20.1B

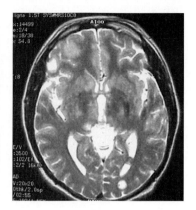

FIG. 20.1C

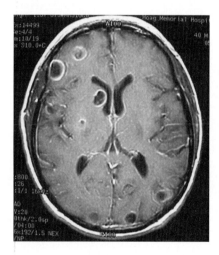

FIG. 20.1D

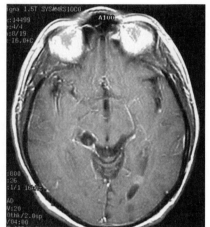

FIG. 20.1E

CLINICAL HISTORY

A 40-year-old man with seizure disorder.

FINDINGS

Sagittal T1-weighted acquisition (Fig. 20.1A) demonstrates multiple well-defined and rounded low signal lesions scattered throughout the supratentorial brain parenchyma. Several lesions have a small punctate focus of intermediate signal material within them. Most of the lesions lie within the cortex with some deep gray matter lesions also present. Axial T2-weighted images (Fig. 20.1B and C) show these lesions to be hyperintense. There is no significant perifocal edema. Note the lesion within the occipital horn of the left lateral ventricle. Postcontrast images (Fig. 20.1D and E) show most of the lesions to peripherally enhance. An enhancing lesion is also identified within the quadrigeminal plate cistern on the right.

DIAGNOSIS

Neurocysticercosis.

DISCUSSION

Neurocysticercosis is the most common parasitic central nervous system (CNS) infection in the world. The infection is caused by the *Taenia solium* parasite (pork tapeworm). This parasite is endemic in Asia, Central and South America, Africa, and Mexico. Its incidence is rapidly increasing in North America. The larval form of the tapeworm is the agent responsible for CNS cysticercosis. Humans are the definitive host of the tapeworm *T. solium* and usually harbor the adult tapeworm in the small intestine as an asymptomatic infestation. Eggs are shed by the definitive host (humans) in the feces and are then ingested (usually via contaminated water or food) by the intermediate host (typically pigs or humans). Once in the intestine, the eggs release oncospheres, the primary larvae. The primary larvae bore through the intestinal wall and enter the blood stream. There is then hematogenous spread to neural, muscular, and ocular tissues. When pigs are the intermediate host, neurocysticercosis is contracted by humans via the ingestion of oncospheres (primary larvae) in poorly cooked pork. Once in the brain, oncospheres transform into secondary larvae: the cysticerci. Cysticerci are ovoid paralytic cysts, which consist of a focal rounded collection of clear fluid (rarely greater than 1.5 cm) with central invaginated scolex or larval head. The CNS is involved in 60% to 90% of patients with cysticercosis. The identification of these cysticerci on neuroimaging is virtually pathognomonic of this disease. The cyst evokes little host reaction as long as it remains intact. Once implanted, these parasitic cysts can lie dormant for years. Eventually, however, the larvae die and there is an acute inflammatory reaction related to degeneration of the cyst, granulation tissue, and scar formation. It is this marked host response following larval death that results in the morbidity associated with neurocysticercosis. In the final stage, the cyst usually calcifies.

The brain parenchyma is the most commonly affected site in neurocysticercosis (more than 50%). Lesions are typically found at the corticomedullary junction. Intraventricular cysticercosis is found in 20% to 50% of cases. The fourth ventricle is the most common site. Neurocysticercosis is rarely isolated to the subarachnoid space (seen in only 10% of cases). More than one anatomic site is usually involved.

Clinically, patients typically present with seizures (50% to 70%), headache, signs of intracranial hypertension, and/or focal neurological deficit.

On imaging, there are four patterns of disease that reflect the pathology of, and host response to, neurocysticercosis. These include the vesicular, colloidal vesicular, granular nodular, and nodular calcified stage. During the first stage (vesicular stage), the secondary larva (cysticercus) consists of a thin capsule surrounding a viable larva and its fluid-containing bladder. On neuroimaging, the cysticercus appears as a round cerebrospinal fluid (CSF) signal cyst with an intermediate signal eccentric nodule that represents the scolex (or larval head). This imaging feature is nicely demonstrated in this case. The scolex is often best seen on fluid-attenuated inversion-recovery or proton density acquisition. Perifocal edema and enhancement are extremely rare. The colloidal vesicular stage represents the death and degeneration of the larva, prompting an acute inflammatory response. The host forms a thickened fibrous capsule with resultant parenchymal edema with ring (two thirds of cases) or nodular-type enhancement. Cyst fluid is hyperintense/hyperdense on MRI and CT, respectively. During the granular nodular stage, the cyst retracts and forms a nodule, which will eventually calcify. Occasionally, the scolex is calcified at this stage. The cysts are isodense on CT with or without central calcification. The lesion is typically isointense on T1-weighted images and isointense to hypointense on T2-weighted acquisition. Nodular or micro ring enhancement is common at this stage, suggestive of granuloma. Perifocal edema persists. The final stage is the nodular calcified stage in which the lesion has shrunk and become mineralized. On CT, there are single or multiple calcified nodules. On MRI, the lesions are hypointense on all pulse sequences. Lesions are most conspicuous on gradient echo acquisition. Typically, there is little or no edema or enhancement in this stage. Enhancement of calcified nodules in the nodular calcified stage has, however, been reported. The presence of parenchymal calcifications on CT studies has been identified as the only independent factor directly related to seizure recurrence after cysticidal therapy. The presence of persistent enhancement of calcified lesions may be an additional risk factor for posttreatment seizures.

Intraventricular cysticercosis accounts for 20% to 50% of neurocysticercosis. As in the parenchymal form, the status of the larva determines the imaging findings. A dying intraventricular larva results in ventriculitis. Most often, intraventricular cysts are unattached and freely mobile. As a result, they can cause intermittent or positional obstruction of the ventricular system with potential for sudden death, highlighting the importance of their detection. In contradistinction to parenchymal cysts, intraventricular cysts very rarely calcify. On MRI, the cyst wall, scolex, and subependymal reaction are readily seen.

In cisternal neurocysticercosis, the subarachnoid space and meninges are involved. It is rare as an isolated finding and is frequently associated with parenchymal disease. Hydrocephalus is often present, either obstructive or related to basal arachnoiditis. A racemose form of subarachnoid cysticercosis features a multiloculated cyst measuring several centimeters in size. They usually occur in the basal cistern or cerebellopontine angle and can simulate low-density tumors. Subarachnoid cysticerci are unique in that they lack a scolex.

Involvement of the spinal canal (shown in Case 52) is thought to be the result of CSF dissemination of the larvae via the subarachnoid space from the cerebrum. Spinal cysticercosis presents as intradural extramedullary cysts and/or arachnoiditis. Intramedullary cysticercosis is extremely rare but has been reported.

SUGGESTED READING

Noujaim SE, Rossi MD, Rao SK, et al. CT and MR imaging of neurocysticercosis. *AJR* 1999;173:1,485–1,490.

Osborn AG. Infections of the brain and its linings. In: *Diagnostic neuroradiology,* 1st ed. St. Louis: Mosby, 1994:708–709.

Rhee RS, Kumasaki DY, Sarwar M, et al. MR imaging of intraventricular cysticercosis. *JCAT* 1987;11(4):598–601.

Sheth TN, Pilon L, Keystone J, et al. Persistent MR contrast enhancement of calcified neurocysticercosis lesions. *AJNR* 1998;19:79–82.

Suss RA, Maravilla KR, Thompson J. MR imaging of intracranial cysticercosis: comparison with CT and anatomopathologic features. *AJNR* 1986;7:235–242.

Zee C, Segall HD, Boswell W, et al. MR imaging of neurocysticercosis. *JCAT* 1988;12(6):927–934.

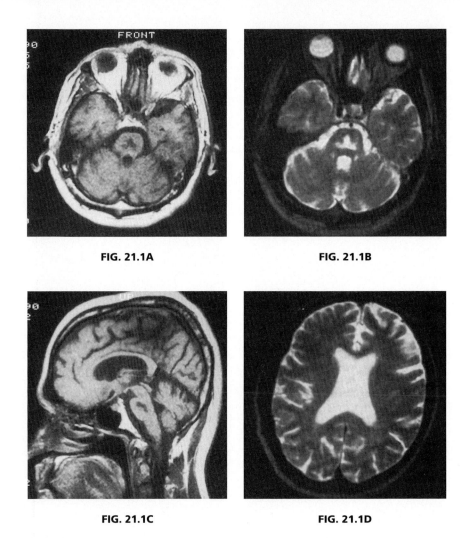

FIG. 21.1A

FIG. 21.1B

FIG. 21.1C

FIG. 21.1D

CLINICAL HISTORY

A 44-year-old alcoholic man recently recovered from a long period of coma following a major binge.

FINDINGS

Axial T1-weighted and T2-weighted images through the pons (Fig. 21.1A–C) demonstrate abnormal signal intensity in the mid pons in the shape of an upside-down butterfly or bat. A section through the lateral ventricles (Fig. 21.1D) demonstrates prominence of the lateral ventricles and sulci. *Submitted by William G. Bradley, M.D., Ph.D., F.A.C.R., Senior Editor, Long Beach Memorial Medical Center, Long Beach, California.*

DIAGNOSIS

Central pontine myelinolysis.

DISCUSSION

Central pontine myelinolysis is most commonly seen in alcoholics presenting with hyponatremia, which is too rapidly corrected in the hospital. Because the process can also involve the thalamus and other extrapontine locations, the newer term "osmotic myelinolysis" has been suggested. The disease can also be seen in other conditions in which hyponatremia is corrected too rapidly, leading to osmotically driven fluid shifts.

The central location within the pons is classic and leads to a "locked-in" condition in which the patient can receive information but not express himself, thus appearing comatose. This is due to involvement of the reticular formation, which in a sense is the central switchboard of the brain.

While the prominent ventricles and sulci shown in Figure 21.1D could represent atrophy, this is really a pathologic diagnosis that should generally not be made on the basis of these imaging findings. Several conditions such as alcoholism, starvation, and catabolic steroid use can give this appearance at one stage in the disease and then return to normal following treatment.

SUGGESTED READING

Laubenberger J, Schneider B, Ansorge O, et al. Central pontine myelinolysis: clinical presentation and radiologic findings. *Eur Radiol* 1996;6-2:177.

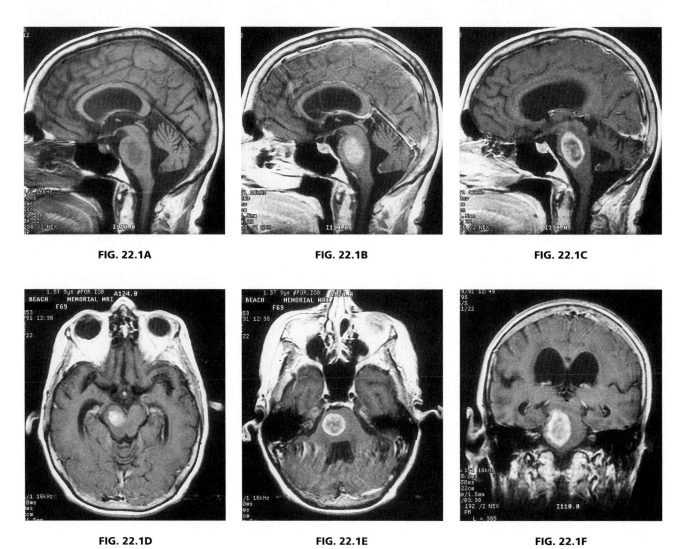

FIG. 22.1A   **FIG. 22.1B**   **FIG. 22.1C**

FIG. 22.1D   **FIG. 22.1E**   **FIG. 22.1F**

CLINICAL HISTORY

A 69-year-old woman with known carcinoma of the lung now presents with worsening left facial palsy, left hemiparesis, and numbness on the left side of her body.

FINDINGS

There is an enhancing ovoid mass in the brainstem, extending from the right cerebral peduncle superiorly into the lower pons inferiorly (Fig. 22.1A–F). The lesion is centrally necrotic and compresses the aqueduct sufficiently (Fig. 22.1B) to cause obstructive hydrocephalus (Fig. 22.1B and F). *Submitted by William G. Bradley, M.D., Ph.D., F.A.C.R., Senior Editor, Long Beach Memorial Medical Center, Long Beach, California.*

DIAGNOSIS

Brainstem metastasis.

DISCUSSION

The differential diagnosis of a single enhancing mass in the brain depends on the patient's age, with patients older than 60 years being more likely to have isolated metastases and those less than 60 being more likely to have gliomas. Depending on the imaging technology used, metastatic disease to the brain presents as an isolated mass 20% to 40% of the time. Eighty percent of all hematogenous metastases to the brain go directly to the parenchyma, as in this case (although this case is unusual in that most isolated metastases involve the anterior circulation due its greater blood flow). Twenty percent of hematogenous metastases go to the leptomeninges. The off-midline position of this metastasis is indicative of the blood supply to the brainstem, i.e., paramedian perforators arising from the basilar artery. (This is the reason brainstem infarctions also tend to have a sharp midline border.) This metastasis is clearly centered on the right side of the brainstem, rather than in the midline.

There is a reasonable correlation between the specific location of lesions in the brainstem and the specific symptoms produced. In this case, the left hemiparesis results from involvement of the right corticospinal tract as it descends through the ventral aspect of the brainstem. The left facial palsy results from involvement of the medial aspect of the cerebral peduncle (Fig. 22.1D), which contains the corticobulbar tract. (Note that the corticobulbar fibers do not cross until they reach the level of the cranial nerve nucleus they innervate.) The numbness on the left side of the body results from involvement of the right medial lemniscus and spinothalamic tract, which carries touch/proprioception and pain/temperature information, respectively.

SUGGESTED READING

Bradley WG. Brainstem: normal anatomy and pathology. In: Stark DD, Bradley WG, eds. *Magnetic resonance imaging,* 3rd ed. St. Louis: Mosby, 1999:1,187–1,208.

Bradley WG. MRI of the brainstem: a practical approach. *Radiology* 1991;179:319–332.

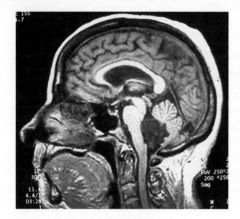

FIG. 23.1A

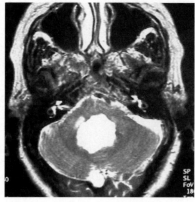

FIG. 23.1B

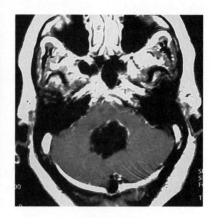

FIG. 23.1C

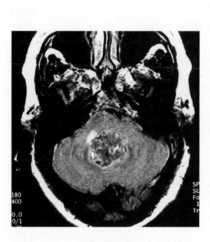

FIG. 23.1D

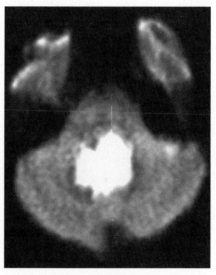

FIG. 23.1E

CLINICAL HISTORY

A 70-year-old woman with history of instability.

FINDINGS

Midline sagittal T1-weighted image (Fig. 23.1A) demonstrates a subtle multilobulated mass in the fourth ventricle. The mass has slightly higher signal than cerebrospinal fluid (CSF). Axial fast spin echo T2-weighted image (Fig. 23.1B) demonstrates diffuse high signal within the lesion with some intermediate signal architecture centrally. Axial postcontrast T1-weighted image (Fig. 23.1C) shows no enhancement of the mass. The mass exhibits heterogeneous signal on the axial fluid-attenuated inversion-recovery (FLAIR) acquisition (Fig. 23.1D), indicative of a solid or semisolid mass. Axial diffusion-weighted image (Fig. 23.1E) shows diffuse high signal within it, indicating limited diffusion further delineating it from CSF.

DIAGNOSIS

Epidermoid.

DISCUSSION

Epidermoid tumors or cysts are slow-growing congenital inclusions, which are derived from tissues of epidermal origin. They are thought to result from the inclusion of epithelium during neural tube closure in the third to fifth week of embryogenesis (or rarely as a result of traumatic or iatrogenic implantation of epidermal elements). They are composed of a wall of simple stratified squamous epithelium with a central collection of desquamative waxy keratin products. Epidermoids represent approximately 0.5% to 1.5% of all intracranial neoplasms. They are usually diagnosed later in life (in the second to fourth decade) because of their slow growth and limited symptomatology. The most common presenting complaints are seizure and headache in supratentorial lesions and cranial nerve dysfunction or vertigo in those below the tentorium. These tumors are extraaxial in location and occur most commonly within the cerebellopontine angle and parasellar regions. Other less common locations include the rhomboid fossa (ventral to the brainstem), ventricles and choroidal fissures, and subfrontal and interhemispheric regions. Fourth ventricular epidermoid tumors (as seen in this case) account for about 16% of epidermoid tumors. Epidermoids are typically located laterally (as opposed to the midline location of dermoid tumors). They grow locally and tend to insinuate themselves into the subarachnoid cisterns and sulci.

On CT, epidermoids are lobulated extraaxial masses, which exhibit low density, like cerebrospinal fluid (CSF). They may be slightly denser than CSF and are rarely hyperdense. There may be internal tumor matrix. Enhancement is typically not seen. On MRI, epidermoids are characteristically equal to or slightly higher in signal than CSF on all pulse sequences. The FLAIR acquisition is one of the most useful sequences in the diagnosis of epidermoid cyst, as they are almost always hyperintense to CSF on this sequence. The importance of evaluating the signal of the mass as compared with CSF is to differentiate epidermoid tumors from simple arachnoid cysts, which will follow CSF signal on all pulse sequences. MRI will often demonstrate internal architecture within epidermoid tumors, another distinguishing feature from arachnoid cyst. Diffusion-weighted imaging is the latest and most promising tool we have in the distinction of these entities. Using the differences in diffusion characteristics between the freely mobile protons within arachnoid cysts and the limited motion within the solid or semisolid matrix of epidermoid cysts, we can make the distinction easily. Epidermoid tumors demonstrate limited diffusion and appear bright on diffusion-weighted images while arachnoid cysts will follow CSF signal and appear dark. Magnetic resonance spectroscopy may also be helpful in the differentiation of these entities. Studies have shown the presence of a lactate peak in epidermoid cysts, whereas arachnoid cysts have minimal lactate on magnetic resonance spectroscopy.

SUGGESTED READING

Aprile I, Iariza F, Lavaroni A, et al. Analysis of cystic intracranial lesions performed with fluid-attenuated inversion-recovery MR imaging. *AJNR* 1999;20(7):1,259–1,267.

Ikushima I, Korogi Y, Hirai T, et al. MR of epidermoids with a variety of pulse sequences. *AJNR* 1997;18(7):1,359–1,363.

Ishikawa M, Kikuchi H, Asato R. MR imaging of the intracranial epidermoid. *Acta Neurochir (Wien)* 1989;101(3-4):108–111.

Kallmes DF, Provenzale JM, Cloft HJ. Typical and atypical MR imaging features of intracranial epidermoid tumors. *AJR* 1997;169(3):883–887.

Panagopoulos KP, el-Azouzim, Chisholm HL, et al. Intracranial epidermoids. A continuing diagnostic challenge. *Arch Neurol* 1990;47(7):813–816.

Poptani H, Gupta RK, Jain VK. Cystic intracranial mass lesions: possible role of in vivo MR spectroscopy in its differential diagnosis. *Magn Reson Imaging* 1995;13(7):1,019–1,029.

Tsuruda JS, Chew WM, Moseley ME, et al. Diffusion-weighted MR imaging of the brain: value of differentiating between extraaxial cysts and epidermoid tumors. *AJR* 1990;155(5):1,059–1,065.

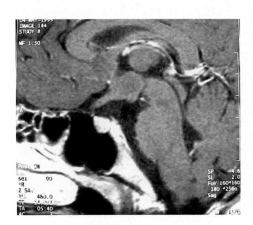

FIG. 24.1A

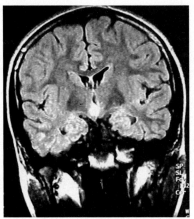

FIG. 24.1B

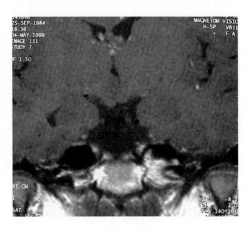

FIG. 24.1C

CLINICAL HISTORY

A 15-year-old girl with history of seizures.

FINDINGS

Sagittal noncontrast T1-weighted acquisition (Fig. 24.1A) demonstrates an isointense mass in the region of the hypothalamus. It lies immediately anterior to the mammillary bodies and posterior to the pituitary stalk. Coronal fluid-attenuated inversion-recovery acquisition (Fig. 24.1B) shows the mass to be hyperintense and arising from the tuber cinereum just to the right of midline. The postcontrast T1-weighted acquisition in the coronal plane (Fig. 24.1C) shows no enhancement.

DIAGNOSIS

Hamartoma of the tuber cinereum.

DISCUSSION

A hamartoma of the tuber cinereum is a congenital non-neoplastic heterotopia made up of disorganized neural tissue that histologically resembles cerebral cortex. It is best known for its association with gelastic seizures (spasmodic or hysteric laughter); however, it more commonly presents as precocious puberty. Very rarely, this lesion is associated with other congenital abnormalities such as callosal agenesis, optic malformations, heterotopias, or microgyria.

On imaging, they appear as a sessile or pedunculated mass attached to the posterior hypothalamus between the pituitary stalk and mamillary bodies. They are homogeneous lesions, isointense to gray matter on T1-weighted images and isointense to slightly hyperintense on proton density and T2-weighted acquisition. Rarely, calcification, fat, or cystic changes have been reported. Contrast enhancement is atypical.

Differential diagnosis includes hypothalamic glioma and craniopharyngioma. Both of these tumors are typically more heterogeneous, enhance, and are not isointense to gray matter on T1-weighted images.

SUGGESTED READING

Boyko OB, Curnes JT, Oakes WJ, et al. Hamartomas of the tuber cinereum: CT, MR, and pathologic findings. *AJNR* 1991;12(2):309–314.

Burton EM, Ball WS Jr, Cronek K, et al. Hamartoma of the tuber cinereum: a comparison of MR and CT findings in four cases. *AJNR* 1989;10(3):497–501.

Hahn FJ, Leibrock LG, Huseman CA, et al. The MR appearance of hypothalamic hamartoma. *Neuroradiology* 1988;30:65–68.

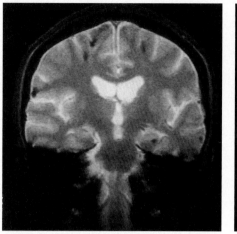 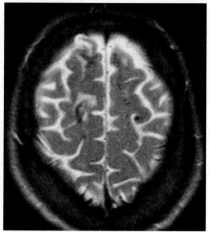

FIG. 25.1A   **FIG. 25.1B**

CLINICAL HISTORY

A 12-year-old boy in a motor vehicle accident now with a Glasgow coma scale score of 12 (without elevated intracranial pressure) after several weeks in the intensive care unit.

FINDINGS

Multiple areas of low-signal intensity are noted on coronal and axial gradient echo image (Fig. 25.1A) and axial T2-weighted conventional spin echo image (Fig. 25.1B) at the gray-white junction peripherally. *Submitted by William G. Bradley, M.D., Ph.D., F.A.C.R., Senior Editor, Long Beach Memorial Medical Center, Long Beach, California.*

DIAGNOSIS

Hemorrhagic shear injury.

DISCUSSION

Shear injury, or "diffuse axonal injury," results from rotatory head trauma. As the rotating skull hits the nonrotating windshield during a motor vehicle accident, the brain continues to turn and shears at points of differing Young modulus or stiffness. Typically, these areas are the gray-white junction, the posterior corpus callosum, the posterior limb of the internal capsule, and the posterolateral upper brainstem.

Shear injury can be either hemorrhagic or bland. When hemorrhagic, punctate hyperdensity may be seen on CT upon admission. MRI in the acute phase will demonstrate rounded areas of hypodensity on T2-weighted images corresponding to the intracellular deoxyhemoglobin. This is best seen on T2-weighted gradient echo images, next best seen on T2-weighted spin echo, and least well seen on T2-weighted fast spin echo (as the closely spaced 180 degree pulses tend to minimize diffusion-meditated dephasing effects from magnetic susceptibility).

Clinically, these patients present with a decreased Glasgow coma scale score for long periods, reflecting disruption of white matter tracts. While most cases of diffuse axonal injury will appear hemorrhagic on high field systems, many appear more bland, i.e., less hemorrhagic, on lower field systems.

SUGGESTED READING

Evans SJJ, Gean AD. Craniocerebral trauma. In: Stark DD, Bradley WG, eds. *Magnetic resonance imaging,* 3rd ed. St. Louis: Mosby, 1999:1,347–1,360.

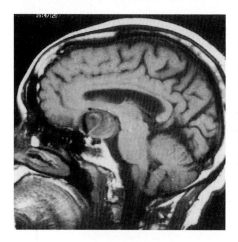

FIG. 26.1A

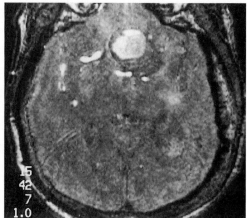

FIG. 26.1B

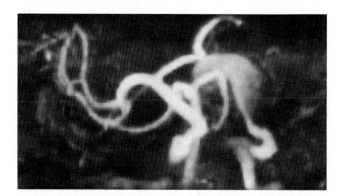

FIG. 26.1C

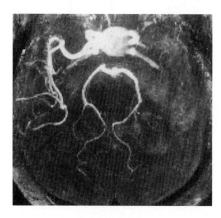

FIG. 26.1D

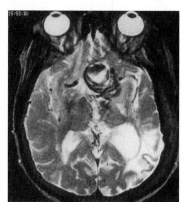

FIG. 26.1E

CLINICAL HISTORY

A 32-year-old woman presenting with headaches progressing to aphasia and right hemiparesis.

FINDINGS

A heterogeneous suprasellar mass (Fig. 26.1A) is noted with selected views from magnetic resonance angiograms (MRAs) (Fig. 26.1B–D). T2-weighted axial images of the brain demonstrate hyperintensity in the left temporal lobe (Fig. 26.1E). *Submitted by William G. Bradley, M.D., Ph.D., F.A.C.R., Senior Editor, Long Beach Memorial Medical Center, Long Beach, California.*

DIAGNOSES

(i) Giant intracranial aneurysm and (ii) left middle cerebral artery (MCA) infarction.

DISCUSSION

A giant intracranial aneurysm is defined on the basis of a diameter greater than 2.5 cm. This one arises from the distal left MCA and contains a turbulent jet (low signal) arising from the aneurysm's neck, surrounded by heterogeneous low-signal intensity that is less than that of adjacent brain on the sagittal T1-weighted image (Fig. 26.1A). Before the availability of MRA, the nature of the low signal within the aneurysm dome was debated: Was it slowing flowing blood or clot? By comparing the source image from the MRA (Fig. 26B) to the T1-weighted image (Fig. 26.1A), the higher signal on the source image indicates slow flow. (High signal due to clot from methemoglobin would have also been bright on the T1-weighted image.) Figure 26.1C was formed from 64 source images, and subjected to a maximum intensity projection (MIP) algorithm. The aneurysm is viewed from behind and demonstrates a fundamental difference between MRA and catheter angiography. The highest signal on the MRA comes from areas of rapid flow, i.e., the turbulent jet coming from the neck, while areas of slower flow within the aneurysm dome produce less signal. With contrast-based techniques such as catheter angiography and CT angiography, the signal is based more on the patent lumen than on flow per se.

The left MCA cutoff in Figure 26.1D and the associated high signal in the left MCA distribution (Fig. 26.1E) represents an infarct. In general, this could be due to vascular spasm secondary to subarachnoid hemorrhage (not seen here) or mass effect or changing orientation of the aneurysm as it expands near the origin of the left middle cerebral artery. If the left MCA originates from the dome of the aneurysm, natural thrombosis (or that induced by coiling or clipping) can also lead to secondary infarcts.

SUGGESTED READING

Litt A, Maltin EP. Cerebrovascular abnormalities. In: Stark DD, Bradley WG, eds. *Magnetic resonance imaging,* 3rd ed. St. Louis: Mosby, 1999:1,317–1,328.

Masarayk TJ, Perl J, et al. Magnetic resonance angiography: neuroradiological applications. In: Stark DD, Bradley WG, eds. *Magnetic resonance imaging,* 3rd ed. St. Louis: Mosby, 1999:1,277–1,316.

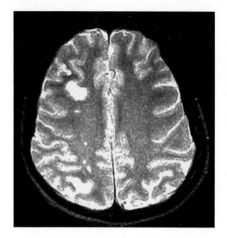

FIG. 27.1A

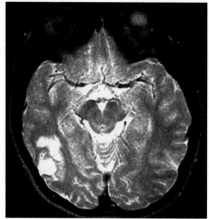

FIG. 27.1B

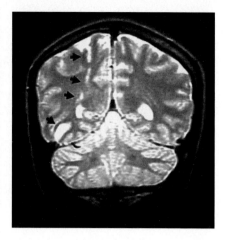

FIG. 27.1C

CLINICAL HISTORY

A 30-year-old woman with left-sided weakness.

FINDINGS

Axial and coronal T2-weighted images (Fig. 27.1A–C) show regions of abnormal high signal within the cortex, subcortical, and deep white matter of the right frontal, parietal, and posterior temporal lobes. The regions of signal abnormality lie at the junction between the vascular territories of the anterior and middle and the posterior and middle cerebral arteries, as well as in the distribution of the deep perforating branches.

DIAGNOSIS

Watershed infarct.

DISCUSSION

The distribution of ischemia in the watershed region is typically caused by diminished perfusion pressure within the ipsilateral carotid artery, as opposed to an embolic event (which tends to involve a selected gray matter territory supplied by one of the branch vessels, as well as the underlying white matter). The "watershed" represents the distal-most supply of the smallest branches and thus lies at the junctional zone between the major cortical branches (the anterior, middle, and posterior cerebral arteries). Also, the distal-most distribution of the deep perforating arteries is involved, thus producing deep white matter lesions that typically conform to a semilunar morphology when connecting the abnormal foci.

Causes of watershed infarction in the elderly patient include cardiac output problems (e.g., arrhythmia) superimposed on carotid occlusive disease or sudden occlusion of the internal carotid artery (without embolization), particularly when superimposed on contralateral carotid disease or incompleteness of the circle of Willis (congenital hypoplasia or aplasia of the anterior A1 segment of the anterior communicating artery). In younger patients, dissection of the carotid artery (without embolization) should also be considered as a potential cause.

SUGGESTED READING

Evrard S, Wolmant F, Le Coz P, et al. Watershed cerebral infarcts: retrospective study of 24 cases. *Neurol Res* 1992;14:97–99.

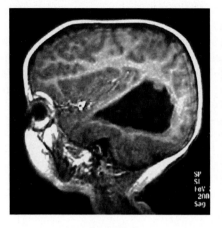

FIG. 28.1A

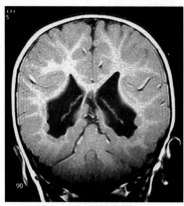

FIG. 28.1B

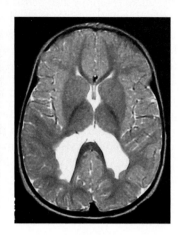

FIG. 28.1C

CLINICAL HISTORY

A 2-year-old girl with a seizure disorder.

FINDINGS

Sagittal and coronal noncontrast T1-weighted images (Fig. 28.1A and B) and axial T2-weighted images (Fig. 28.1C) demonstrate multiple small nodules along the walls of the lateral ventricles bilaterally. These are most conspicuous within the atria and temporal horns. The nodules are isointense to gray matter on both sequences. There is asymmetric dilation of the atria and temporal horns of the lateral ventricles. The gyral and sulcar patterns are normal. There are no regions of abnormal signal within the cortex or deep white matter.

DIAGNOSIS

Nodular heterotopia.

DISCUSSION

Gray matter heterotopia is one entity in a spectrum of congenital abnormalities known as the "neuronal migrational disorders" (NMDs). NMDs accounted for 4.3% of all epilepsy patients referred for MRI in one study. Although they are congenital disorders, the onset of seizures is surprisingly late, often after 10 years of age. It is uncertain if heterotopic gray matter is the actual cause of seizures or if it is a marker of an abnormal process that results in seizure activity.

NMDs range from gray matter heterotopias to sulcar anomalies depending on the time and extent of migration arrest. Heterotopia represents the earliest migrational arrest in which a collection of normal gray matter is found in an abnormal location. Nodular heterotopia is a focus or foci of gray matter that never migrates and is usually found in the subependymal region. Laminar or band heterotopia occurs when there is diffuse arrest of neuronal migration resulting in a layer of ectopic gray matter between the ventricles and cortex. Occasionally, heterotopia presents as a large mass of dysplastic gray matter involving part or all of a cerebral hemisphere. Heterotopia may be an isolated finding or associated with other sulcar anomalies (e.g., pachygyria or polymicrogyria) and dysplasias (e.g., corpus callosum).

Because MRI is superior to CT in differentiating gray and white matter, it is the modality of choice in imaging NMDs. Nodular heterotopia appears as multiple confluent subependymal masses, which are identical in signal intensity to gray matter on all pulse sequences. There is no enhancement following contrast. The characteristic signal intensity helps to differentiate this entity from the subependymal nodules seen in tuberous sclerosis, which demonstrate high signal on T2-weighted acquisition and can enhance (see Case 46). Band heterotopia features a thick symmetric band of gray matter within the centrum semiovale, interposed between the ventricles and cortex. There is typically a thin layer of residual normal white matter between the heterotopic gray matter and normal overlying cortex (see Case 75).

This case nicely demonstrates the nodular form of gray matter heterotopia.

SUGGESTED READING

Barkovich AJ, Kjos BO. Gray matter heterotopia: MR characteristics and correlation with developmental and neurologic manifestations. *Radiology* 1992;182(2):493–499.

Brodtkorb E, Nilsen G, Smevik O, et al. Epilepsy and abnormalities of neuronal migration: MRI and clinical aspects. *Acta Neurol Scand* 1992;86:24–32.

Canapicchi R, Padolecchia R, Puglioli M, et al. Heterotopic gray matter. Neuroradiological aspects and clinical correlation. *J Neuroradiol* 1990;17(4):277–287.

Hayden SA, Davis KA, Stears JC, et al. MR imaging of heterotopic gray matter. *JCAT* 1987;11(5):878–879.

Smith AS, Weinstein MA, Quencer RM, et al. Association of heterotopic gray matter with seizures: MR imaging. Work in progress. *Radiology* 1988;168(1):195–198.

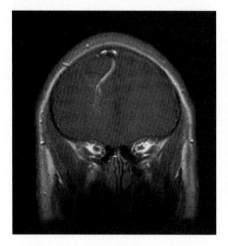

FIG. 29.1A

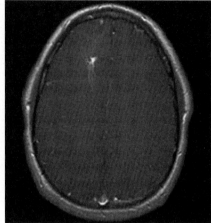

FIG. 29.1B

CLINICAL HISTORY

A 17-year-old boy with headaches. Recent head trauma while playing football.

FINDINGS

Coronal and axial T1-weighted images after intravenous gadolinium-DTPA contrast administration (Fig. 29.1A and B) demonstrate enhancing radially oriented subcortical veins within the right frontal lobe that drain into a single large transcortical vein. *Submitted by Alan D.S. Chan, M.D., and William G. Bradley, M.D., Ph.D., F.A.C.R., Senior Editor, Long Beach Memorial Medical Center, Long Beach, California.*

DIAGNOSIS

Venous angioma or developmental venous anomaly.

DISCUSSION

Developmental venous anomalies or venous malformations are considered to be incidental vascular malformations of venous drainage. They consist of multiple, dilated, radially oriented subcortical veins that converge and drain into a single large transcortical vein. Thus, they resemble the characteristic "Medusa's head" configuration. No arteriovenous shunting is present. They may, although rarely, cause headaches, focal neurological deficits, or seizures. There may be narrowing of the draining vein near its site of drainage into a dural venous sinus, which can result in venous hypertension, thrombosis, or hemorrhage. If chronic venous hypertension is present, venous ischemia may develop. The frontal lobes are the most common locations. However, they can also be located in the brainstem or cerebellum where they have a slightly increased incidence of hemorrhage.

SUGGESTED READING

Gledhill K, Moor KR, Jacobs JM, et al. Cerebrovascular disease. In: Orrison WW, ed. *Neuroimaging.* Philadelphia: WB Saunders, 2000.

Meyers PM, Halbach VV, Barkovich AJ. Anomalies of cerebral vasculature: diagnostic and endovascular considerations. In: Barkovich AJ, ed. *Pediatric neuroimaging.* Philadelphia: Lippincott Williams & Wilkins, 2000.

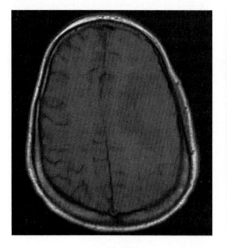

FIG. 30.1A

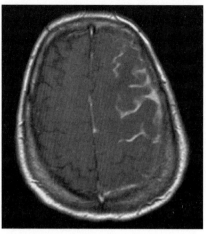

FIG. 30.1B

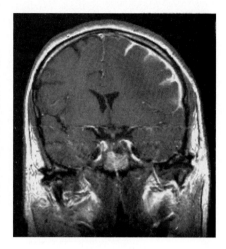

FIG. 30.1C

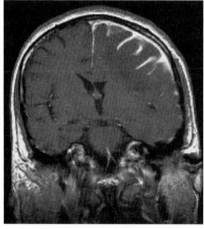

FIG. 30.1D

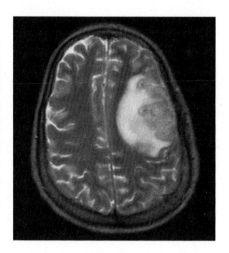

FIG. 30.1E

CLINICAL HISTORY

A 37-year-old man with history of seizures and Crohn disease now presents with progressive aphasia.

FINDINGS

Axial and coronal T1-weighted images after intravenous gadolinium-DTPA contrast administration (Figs. 30.1B–D) demonstrate thick leptomeningeal enhancement over the left frontal lobe. In addition, within the left frontal lobe, there is an indistinct hypointense area on the T1-weighted images (Fig. 30.1A–D) and a hyperintense area on the T2-weighted image (Fig. 30.1E) representing a significant amount of vasogenic edema. As a result, there is mass effect upon the left lateral ventricle and mild subfalcial herniation. *Submitted by Alan D.S. Chan, M.D., and William G. Bradley, M.D., Ph.D., F.A.C.R., Senior Editor, Long Beach Memorial Medical Center, Long Beach, California.*

DIAGNOSIS

Cerebritis.

DISCUSSION

Cerebritis is described as acute inflammation within the brain parenchyma. It can be caused by hematogenous dissemination, direct extension, and in the case of trauma or surgery, penetration of infectious pathogens such as bacteria, viruses, and fungi. Four stages of cerebral abscess formation have been described. Early cerebritis usually occurs within the first few days following an infection. During this stage, sulcal effacement, vasogenic edema, patchy areas of necrosis, petechial hemorrhage, and leptomeningeal enhancement may be demonstrated. During the late stage of cerebritis and early capsule formation stage, typically 4 to 14 days after the infection, a well-defined central necrotic core with an enhancing rim of inflammatory tissue can be seen. During the late capsule formation stage, which occurs more than 2 weeks after the initial infection, a thick collagenous capsule develops around a necrotic core, which is decreasing in size. Surrounding gliosis is also present.

SUGGESTED READING

Grossman RI, Yousem DM. *Neuroradiology: the requisites.* St. Louis: Mosby, 1994.
Sze G. Infection and inflammation. In: Stark DD, Bradley WG, eds. *Magnetic resonance imaging,* 3rd ed. St. Louis: Mosby, 1999:1,361–1,378.

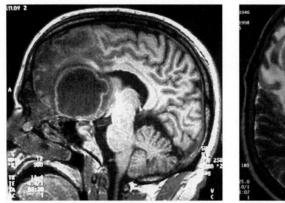

FIG. 31.1A

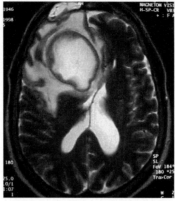

FIG. 31.1B

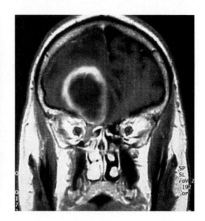

FIG. 31.1C

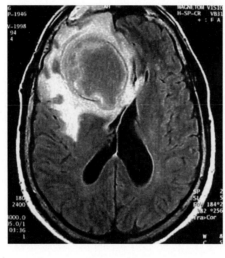

FIG. 31.1D

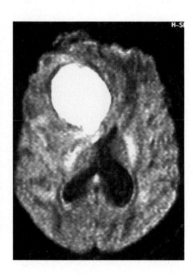

FIG. 31.1E

CLINICAL HISTORY

A 52-year-old man with recent mental status change and fever.

FINDINGS

Sagittal T1-weighted and axial T2-weighted images (Fig. 31.1A and B) demonstrate a large well-circumscribed mass within the right frontal lobe. This lesion is hypointense on T1-weighted images and hyperintense on T2-weighted images. There is a very well defined rim of intermediate signal material on the T1-weighted image, which is of low signal on the T2-weighted acquisition. There is a significant amount of perifocal edema with shift of the midline structures toward the left. Also note abnormal tissue within the right frontal sinus and bilateral ethmoid sinus consistent with sinusitis. Following intravenous contrast (Fig. 31.1C), there is intense peripheral enhancement of the parenchymal mass. Note extension of this process into the subfrontal region and along the cribriform plate on the right. Fluid-attenuated inversion-recovery acquisition (Fig. 31.1D) demonstrates a large hypointense mass with surrounding high signal consistent with edema. Diffusion-weighted images (Fig. 31.1E) show very high signal within the center of this mass consistent with restricted diffusion.

DIAGNOSIS

Frontal and ethmoid sinusitis with large cerebral abscess.

DISCUSSION

Intracranial abscess is the last stage in the evolution of brain parenchymal infection. The stages of abscess formation are as follows: early cerebritis, late cerebritis, early capsule formation, and late capsule formation (mature abscess). The imaging features of these stages reflect the underlying pathophysiology of abscess formation.

The most common route of intracranial infection is via hematogenous spread. Mastoid and sinus infections, as seen in this case, spread intracranially through retrograde thrombophlebitis. Empyema and/or meningitis may precede parenchymal involvement. A congenital or acquired dermal sinus is a less common source of intracranial infection. Most cerebral abscesses are pyogenic or bacterial in origin. The organisms most frequently implicated are streptococci and staphylococci. Gram-negative organisms are becoming a more common cause. Less commonly, mycobacterial and fungal disease cause cerebral abscesses. Bacterial intracranial infections most commonly affect the adult population. Patients with acquired immunodeficiency syndrome rarely develop pyogenic abscesses, although opportunistic infections are common.

Intracranial abscesses are most frequently found in the frontal and parietal lobes, usually at the corticomedullary junction. Less than 15% occur in the posterior fossa.

The early cerebritis phase occurs in the first 3 to 5 days. It consists of focal, but not yet localized, parenchymal infection. At imaging, MRI demonstrates an ill-defined subcortical hyperintense region on T2-weighted images. There may be poorly defined enhancement following contrast. In the late cerebritis phase (day 4 to 14), the infection becomes more circumscribed with regions of central necrosis. There is a thick irregular isointense to hyperintense rim on T1-weighted images, which is characteristically isointense to hypointense on T2-weighted images. Central necrotic areas are hyperintense on long TE scans and there is nearly always perifocal edema. Intense ring enhancement is seen following contrast. The early capsule stage begins at about 2 weeks; the late capsule stage can persist for weeks to months. The capsule is composed of collagen and reticulin. The central core consists of liquefied necrotic and inflammatory debris. The mature abscess appears as a thin-walled, well-defined cystic mass with a hypointense rim on T2-weighted images, and an isointense to hyperintense rim on T1-weighted images persists. It is easily identified on noncontrast scans. The capsule is classically described (50% of cases) as being thinner along its deep (ventricular) margin. As the abscess matures, mass effect and perifocal edema improve. Smaller "daughter abscesses" within the adjacent parenchyma are common. In the late phase, as the abscess heals, the abscess cavity shrinks. Ring enhancement can persist for months—long after the patient has clinically improved.

Complications of cerebral abscess include ventriculitis, choroid plexitis, and purulent leptomeningitis.

Differential diagnosis for a ring-enhancing intracerebral mass is extensive. Cystic or centrally necrotic primary neoplasms, metastatic brain tumor, granuloma, resolving hematoma, and infarct can all resemble cerebral abscess based on neuroimaging, but their enhancing margin tends to be less uniform and discrete. Less common entities in the differential diagnosis include thrombosed vascular malformation or aneurysm and demyelinating disease. Recent advances in diffusion-weighted MRI and magnetic resonance spectroscopy (MRS) have proved useful in differentiating these diagnoses. Abscess typically demonstrates high signal on diffusion-weighted imaging with markedly decreased apparent diffusion coefficient, whereas necrotic tumor will appear hypointense on diffusion-weighted imaging. On MRS, abscesses reveal lactate and amino acid peaks in all patients regardless of the time of spectral acquisition relative to initiation of treatment. Acetate and pyruvate may also be present but usually disappear a week following treatment onset. Amino acids and acetate are not typically found in neoplasm.

SUGGESTED READING

Desprechins B, Stadnik T, Koerts G, et al. Use of diffusion weighted MR imaging in differential diagnosis between intracerebral necrotic tumor and cerebral abscess. *AJNR* 1999;20(7):1,252–1,257.

Dev R, Gupta RU, Poptani H, et al. Role of in vivo proton MR spectroscopy in the diagnosis and management of brain abscesses. *Neurosurgery* 1998;42(1):37–42.

Haimes AB, Zimmerman RD, Morgello S, et al. MR imaging of brain abscess. *AJR* 1989;152(5):1,073–1,085.

Kim YJ, Chang KH, Song IC, et al. Brain abscess and necrotic or cystic tumor: discrimination with signal intensity on diffusion weighted magnetic resonance imaging. *AJR* 1998;17(6):1,490–1,497.

Martinez-Perezi E, Moreno A, Alonso J, et al. Diagnosis of brain abscess by MR spectroscopy: report of two cases. *J Neurosurg* 1997;86(4):708–713.

Osborn AG. Infections of the brain and its linings. In: *Diagnostic neuroradiology,* 1st ed. St. Louis: Mosby, 1994;688–694.

Yang SY, Zhao CS. Review of 40 patients with brain abscess. *Surg Neurol* 1993;39(4):290–296.

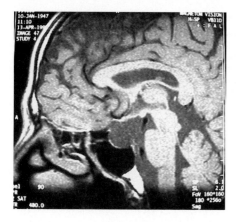

FIG. 32.1A

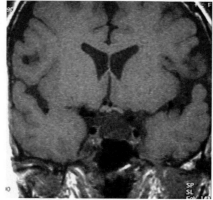

FIG. 32.1B

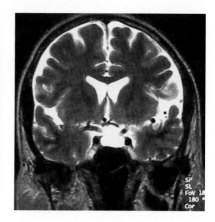

FIG. 32.1C

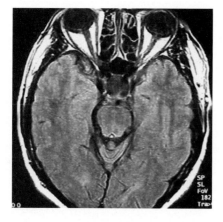

FIG. 32.1D

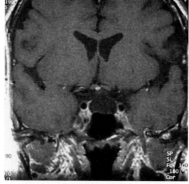

FIG. 32.1E

CLINICAL HISTORY

A 52-year-old man with visual disturbance.

FINDINGS

Sagittal and coronal noncontrast T1-weighted images (Fig. 32.1A and B) demonstrate a large cystic mass within the sella turcica, which is isointense to cerebrospinal fluid (CSF). There is flattening of the pituitary gland along the floor of the sella, as well as enlargement of the sella. Additionally, there is mass effect upon the undersurface of the optic chiasm with some superior displacement. Coronal T2-weighted image (Fig. 32.1C) demonstrates a homogeneous, hyperintense lesion within the sella, again isointense with CSF. Axial fluid-attenuated inversion-recovery acquisition (Fig. 32.1D) shows the lesion to be hypointense, following CSF signal. Following intravenous contrast (Fig. 32.1E), there is no enhancement. Note displacement of the infundibulum toward the right.

DIAGNOSIS

Intrasellar arachnoid cyst.

DISCUSSION

Arachnoid cysts can be acquired secondary to an inflammatory reaction in the subarachnoid space related to meningitis, head trauma, primary subarachnoid hemorrhage, or extraaxial brain tumors. A large number, however, are congenital. These cysts account for 1% of all intracranial masses, with most occurring in the middle fossa. Other possible locations include the frontal convexity region and basal cisterns (i.e., suprasellar and quadrigeminal cisterns as well as foramen magnum region). They can also be intraventricular or intrasellar. Suprasellar arachnoid cysts, as seen in this case, account for approximately 15% of intracranial arachnoid cysts. They are frequently asymptomatic but can cause mass-related symptoms or hydrocephalus. Suprasellar arachnoid cysts can present with visual disturbance and cranial neuropathies.

Imaging demonstrates a well-defined mass that is isodense and isointense to CSF on CT and all MRI pulse sequences. There is often displacement and compression of the adjacent third ventricle. Typically, the cyst has no internal architecture and does not calcify or enhance. Intracystic hemorrhage has been reported but is not common.

Differential diagnostic possibilities for a suprasellar cystic mass include a Rathke cleft cyst and epidermoid cyst. Although difficult to differentiate on CT, neither of these lesions follow CSF signal on all MRI pulse sequences. A Rathke cleft cyst usually contains proteinaceous material, which will cause T1 and T2 shortening. Epidermoid cysts are actually solid/semisolid tumors and are slightly higher in signal than CSF on T1-weighted, T2-weighted, and particularly proton density–weighted images. An internal architecture can often be identified. Diffusion-weighted imaging can also be helpful in differentiating these lesions (see Case 23). Cystic craniopharyngiomas could also be considered, but these tumors are almost always heterogeneous with foci of calcification, hemorrhage, and enhancement.

SUGGESTED READING

Armstrong EA, Harwood-Nash DC, Hoffman H, et al. Benign suprasellar cysts: the CT approach. *AJNR* 1983;4:163–166.

Basauri L, Selman JM. Intracranial arachnoid cysts. *Child Nerv Syst* 1992;8(2):101–104.

Dhooge C, Govaert P, Martens F, et al. Transventricular endoscopic investigation and treatment of suprasellar arachnoid cysts. *Neuropediatrics* 1992;23:245–247.

Eustace S, Toland J, Stack J. CT and MRI of arachnoid cyst with complicating intracystic and subdural hemorrhage. *JCAT* 1992;16:995–997.

Van Tassel P, Cure JK. Nonneoplastic intracranial cysts and cystic lesions. *Semin Ultrasound Comput Tomogr Magn Reson* 1995;16(3):186–211.

Von Wild K. Arachnoid cysts of the middle cranial fossa. *Neurochirurgia (Stuttg)* 1992;35(6):177–182.

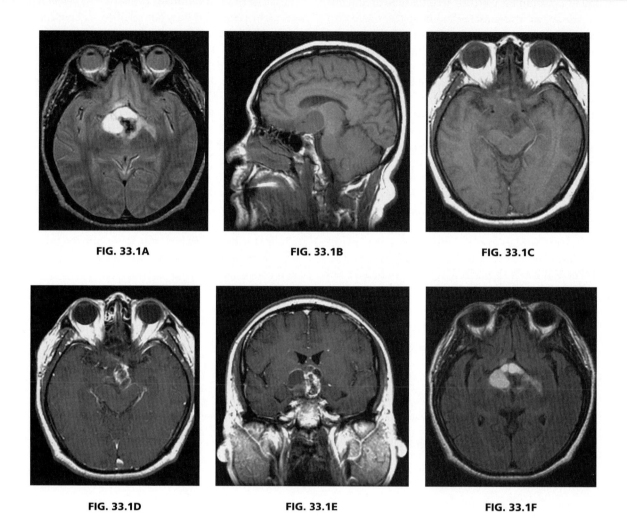

FIG. 33.1A **FIG. 33.1B** **FIG. 33.1C**

FIG. 33.1D **FIG. 33.1E** **FIG. 33.1F**

CLINICAL HISTORY

A 41-year-old man with visual disturbances and headaches.

FINDINGS

Large complex multicystic suprasellar mass. On Figure 33.1C, the focal area of hypointense T2 signal corresponds to calcification on noncontrast head CT (not shown). T1-weighted images (Fig. 33.1B and C) show the cystic components with primarily isointense signal to gray matter. Postcontrast images (Fig. 33.1D and E) demonstrate ring enhancement of cystic components and heterogeneous enhancement of solid components. In addition, edema is seen along the left optic tract (Fig. 33.1A and F). *Submitted by Kathleen M. Flores, M.D., and William G. Bradley, M.D., Ph.D., F.A.C.R., Senior Editor, Long Beach Memorial Medical Center, Long Beach, California.*

DIAGNOSIS

Craniopharyngioma.

DISCUSSION

Craniopharyngiomas are benign neoplasms thought to arise from the pouch of Rathke. They are typically found in the suprasellar cistern in patients of all ages. Over half of these tumors occur in pediatric patients with a smaller peak in the fifth and sixth decades. Although the suprasellar cistern is the most common location for this tumor, it can be found anywhere along the path of the craniopharyngeal duct from the posterior pharynx to the third ventricle.

Characteristic imaging features of craniopharyngiomas include visible cysts and calcification. The cysts usually contain a complex mixture of protein, mucus, cholesterol, blood, and other cellular debris, causing variable signal intensity on MRI. Calcification is a hallmark of craniopharyngiomas, making CT an important part of preoperative imaging historically. In addition, edema can be seen within the optic tracts.

Clinically, patients present with visual symptoms, although symptomatic and nonsymptomatic endocrine abnormalities have also been shown. Treatment is controversial. These tumors are difficult to remove surgically, as they are usually intimately adherent to adjacent neurovascular structures.

SUGGESTED READING

Orrison WW. Extraaxial tumors including pituitary and parasellar. In: Orrison WW, ed. *Neuroimaging.* Philadelphia: WB Saunders, 2000:696–700.

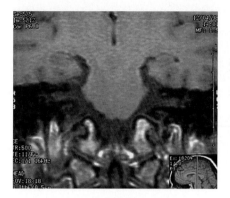

FIG. 34.1A

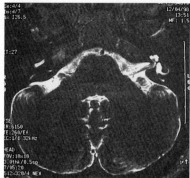

FIG. 34.1B

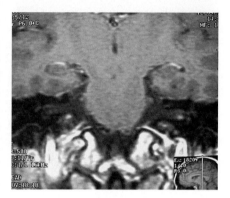

FIG. 34.1C

CLINICAL HISTORY

A 44-year-old woman with left-sided hearing loss.

FINDINGS

Coronal high-resolution targeted images through the internal auditory canals using T1 and fast spin echo T2-weighted images failed to demonstrate abnormality within the internal auditory canals (Fig. 34.1A and B). The seventh and eighth cranial nerves are well seen on the T2-weighted acquisition. No focal mass lesions are identified. Following intravenous contrast (Fig. 34.1C), there is a 1-mm focus of abnormal enhancement along the inferior aspect of the left internal auditory canal.

DIAGNOSIS

Acoustic neuroma.

DISCUSSION

The value of intravenous paramagnetic contrast in the detection of minute acoustic schwannomas is well illustrated in this instance. Although high-resolution imaging with T2-weighted technique is quite sensitive in most cases screened for acoustic tumors, occasionally a minute lesion can be difficult to detect without T1-weighted imaging in combination with intravenous contrast.

On the other hand, the image itself is nonspecific. Fibrosis, hemangioma, viral neuritis (such as that associated with otitic herpes), as well as leptomeningeal spread of disease into the acoustic canal and even neuritis associated with acute disseminated encephalomyelitis of a postvaccinial or postviral type can produce foci of enhancement along the nerves in the internal auditory canal that are indistinguishable from acoustic neuroma. Thus, good clinical history and follow-up are quite important in making a specific diagnosis. Watching the lesion for 2 to 3 months without intervention may be helpful in uncertain cases, as doubling time of acoustic neuroma is 1 to 2 years.

SUGGESTED READING

Allen RW, Harnsberger HR, Shelton C, et al. Low-cost high-resolution fast spin echo MR of acoustic schwannoma: an alternative to enhanced conventional spin echo MR? *AJNR* 1996;17:1,205–1,210.

Gentry LR, Jacoby CG, Turski PA, et al. Cerebellopontine angle-petromastoid mass lesions: comparative study of diagnosis with MR imaging and CT. *Radiology* 1987;162:513–520.

Tien RD, Felsberg GJ, Macfall J. Fast spin echo high-resolution MR imaging of the inner ear. *AJR* 1992;159:395–398.

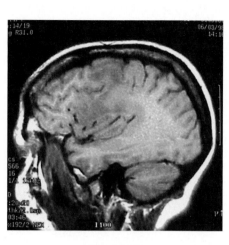

FIG. 35.1A

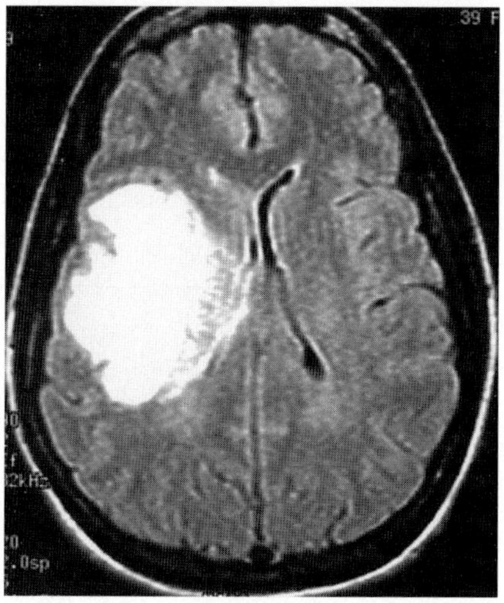

FIG. 35.1B

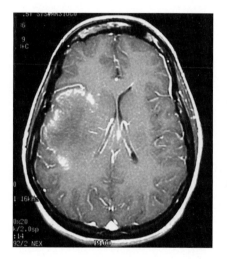

FIG. 35.1C

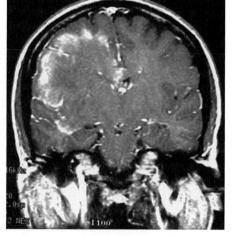

FIG. 35.1D

CLINICAL HISTORY

A 39 year old with acute onset of left-sided weakness.

FINDINGS

Sagittal noncontrast T1-weighted acquisition (Fig. 35.1A) demonstrates poorly defined low signal within the right frontal lobe. Axial fluid-attenuated inversion-recovery images (Fig. 35.1B) show a large region of abnormal high signal involving the subcortical and deep periventricular white matter of the posterior right frontal lobe. There is associated mass effect with effacement of the right lateral ventricle as well as minimal shift of the midline structures toward the left. Postcontrast axial and coronal T1-weighted images (Fig. 35.1C and D) demonstrate poorly defined peripheral enhancement. No other focal intracranial lesions were identified, and the lesion was biopsied.

DIAGNOSIS

Tumefactive acute disseminated encephalomyelitis (ADEM).

DISCUSSION

The acute onset of symptoms initially suggested the diagnosis of infarction in this case, but the fact that the subcortical white matter is predominately involved and that mass effect was present within the first 12 hours made infarction a less likely cause of the imaged lesion. Primary brain tumor is a consideration given the appearance, but these lesions rarely produce acute neurological syndromes. The involvement of the white matter, the relatively young age of the patient, and the very hazy peripheral enhancement suggested tumefactive multiple sclerosis as a consideration, although no other lesions were found. The subsequent workup failed to demonstrate abnormal oligoclonal bands in the cerebrospinal fluid. Biopsy demonstrated a nonspecific demyelinating lesion with no features of infection or neoplasia. Long-term follow-up failed to demonstrate any additional lesions, with the patient recovering over the course of 2 months. She did give a history of recent viral syndrome, prior to the onset of symptoms.

Tumefactive ADEM is unusual, and ADEM typically presents with multifocal white matter lesions and occasionally cranial neuropathy with enhancement of the cranial nerves—the latter helping to distinguish it from multiple sclerosis. Most often, it is seen in childhood following vaccination. It is a monophasic illness without subsequent recurrence (as opposed to multiple sclerosis, which is also thought due to autoimmune etiology). The histology is quite similar to that of multiple sclerosis; thus, occasionally, tumefactive lesions may develop with ADEM, as they do with multiple sclerosis.

SUGGESTED READING

Atlas SW, Grossman RI, Goldberg HI, et al. MR diagnosis of acute disseminated encephalomyelitis. *JCAT* 1986;10:798–801.

Caldmeyer KS, Harris TM, Smith RR, et al. Gadolinium enhancement in acute disseminated encephalomyelitis. *JCAT* 1991;15:673–675.

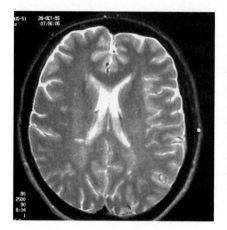

FIG. 36.1A

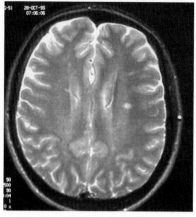

FIG. 36.1B

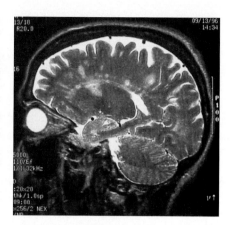

FIG. 36.1C

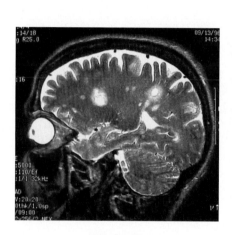

FIG. 36.1D

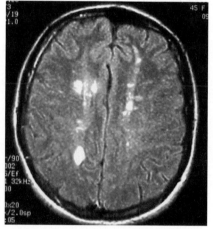

FIG. 36.1E

CLINICAL HISTORY

A 45-year-old woman with right lower extremity weakness as well as numbness and tingling in the upper extremities.

FINDINGS

Axial fast spin echo T2-weighted image (Fig. 36.1A and B) shows several small focal rounded and linear regions of high signal within the deep white matter of both cerebral hemispheres. Note the long axis of the linear lesions lies perpendicular to the long axis of the lateral ventricles. Due to progressive symptoms, the patient had a follow-up study 1 year later. Sagittal fast spin echo T2-weighted images (Fig. 36.1C and D) show a marked increase in the number and size of the lesions, compared with the previous study. Again, most of the lesions are within the deep periventricular white matter and appear as fingerlike projections extending out from the lateral ventricle. Note the large "target" appearance of the lesion within the right parietal lobe. Axial fluid-attenuated inversion-recovery (FLAIR) acquisition (Fig. 36.1E) is useful in making periventricular lesions stand out against the suppressed fluid signal within the ventricles.

DIAGNOSIS

Multiple sclerosis (MS).

DISCUSSION

The etiology of MS is uncertain but is possibly due to an autoimmune-mediated demyelination in genetically susceptible individuals. Symptom onset is usually between the ages of 20 and 40, with a female predominance, particularly when it occurs in children and adolescents. Patients with MS usually present with multifocal neurological deficits. The clinical course is one of prolonged relapsing and remitting disease. Disease can shift into a chronic-progressive phase and rarely a fulminant type (MS of Marburg type), which is associated with a rapid clinical decline with substantial morbidity and mortality.

Pathologically, MS "plaques" appear as edematous white matter lesions. Necrosis and atrophy with cystic change are common in chronic lesions. Hemorrhage and calcification are rare. Microscopically, one sees destruction of myelin and myelin-producing oligodendrocytes with relative sparing of the axon.

The classic imaging feature is multiple ovoid periventricular lesions that are oriented perpendicular to the long axis of the lateral ventricles (seen in 85% of MS patients). This pattern of disease correlates with the propensity of the demyelinating process to occur around subependymal and deep white matter medullary veins. These fingerlike perivascular lesions emanating from the ventricular margin are commonly referred to as "Dawson's fingers." The next most common location for MS plaques is the corpus callosum, typically at the callosal-septal interface. These lesions are most commonly found along the inferior surface of the corpus callosum and are best seen on a sagittal proton density, T2-weighted, or FLAIR image. Involvement of the internal capsule, pons, periaqueductal gray matter, floor of the fourth ventricle, and brachium pontis is common. MS plaques can involve the cortex. MS plaques are typically multifocal; however, a large solitary plaque can occur. Infratentorial lesions (brainstem and cerebellum) are uncommon in adult disease but are frequently seen in children and adolescents with MS.

CT scans are often normal in early MS; therefore, MRI is the imaging modality of choice. When present, MS lesions appear isodense to hypodense on CT with variable enhancement. On MRI, MS plaques are isointense to hypointense on T1-weighted images and hyperintense on T2-weighted and FLAIR acquisition. FLAIR images are particularly helpful in lesion identification because of the suppression of cerebrospinal fluid signal within subjacent ventricles, making periventricular MS lesions more conspicuous. Because there are several etiologies for multiple high-signal periventricular lesions in the brain, some criteria have been established for the MRI diagnosis of MS. These include three or more discrete lesions that are 5 mm or greater in size, a periventricular or callosal-septal distribution, and a compatible clinical history. Identification of the typical oblong perivenular lesions ("Dawson's finger" appearance) is also suggestive of the diagnosis. MS lesions can appear as a "lesion within a lesion" or as a "target" lesion on T1-weighted and proton density images. This imaging appearance is thought to represent a central demyelinating plaque with perifocal edema (which creates the outer "lesion," or halo) or possibly varying degrees of demyelination within a single lesion. In severe disease, the discrete periventricular lesions can become confluent. In approximately 10% of patients with longstanding MS, abnormal hypointense basal ganglia related to iron deposition have been described. Most MS plaques do not enhance following contrast. Enhancement is typically transient and is thought to occur during the active phase of demyelination. Enhancement can be solid or ringlike. A large, solitary enhancing MS plaque can be indistinguishable from tumor or abscess. The large MS plaques are referred to as "tumefactive" MS.

A unique imaging pattern of concentric ri[ ] surrounding an acute MS plaque is known as a "Balo [ ]ntric sclerosis plaque." It is thought to represent free [ ]cals within the macrophage layer at the margin of an acut[ ] demyelinating lesion. The rings are typically multiple and slightly hyperintense on T1-weighted images.

Although MRI is extremely sensitive in the detection of MS plaques, the extent of disease seen on conventional MRI does not correlate well with the clinical status of the patient with regard to disability. Not withstanding the relative correlation between "[ ]tive" disease and contrast enhancement on conventiona[ ] MRI, there is a lack of specificity in the ability to determine the precise biochemical nature of MS lesions using conventional MRI. In this regard, proton magnetic resonance spectroscopy and magnetization transfer magnetic resonance techniques are now being studied and used to better characterize the "activity" of MS lesions in order to monitor treatment response and predict clinical outcome.

SUGGESTED READING

Edwards-Brown MK, Bonnin JM. White matter diseases. In: Atlas SW, ed. *Magnetic resonance imaging of the brain and spine,* 2nd ed. Philadelphia: Lippincott–Raven Publishers, 1996:653–674.

Filippi M. Magnetization transfer imaging to monitor the evolution of individual MS lesions. *Neurology* 1999;53(5, Suppl 3):S18–S22.

Gean-Marton AD, Vezina LG, Marton KI, et al. Abnormal corpus callosum: a sensitive and specific indicator of multiple sclerosis. *Radiology* 1991;180(1):215–221.

Giang DW, Podure KR, Eskin TA, et al. Multiple sclerosis masquerading as a mass lesion. *Neuroradiology* 1992;34:150–154.

Grossman RI, Lenkinski RE, Ramer KN, et al. MR proton spectroscopy in multiple sclerosis. *AJNR* 1992;13:1,535–1,543.

Horowitz AL, Kaplan RD, Grewe G, et al. The ovoid lesions: a new MR observation in patients with multiple sclerosis. *AJNR* 1989;10:303–305.

Nesbit GM, Forbes GS, Scheithauer BW, et al. Multiple sclerosis: histopathologic and MR and/or CT correlation in 37 cases at biopsy and three cases at autopsy. *Radiology* 1991;180:467–474.

Offenbacher H, Fazekas F, Schmitd R, et al. Assessment of MRI criteria for a diagnosis of MS. *Neurology* 1993;43:905–909.

Osborn AG, Harnsberger HR, Smoker WRK, et al. Multiple sclerosis in adolescents: CT and MR findings. *AJNR* 1990;11:489–494.

Powell T, Sussman JG, Davies-Jones GAB. MR imaging in acute multiple sclerosis: ring-like appearance in plaques suggesting the presence of paramagnetic free radicals. *AJNR* 1992;13:1,544–1,546.

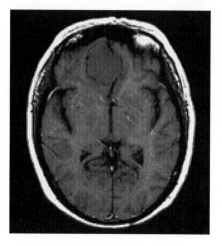
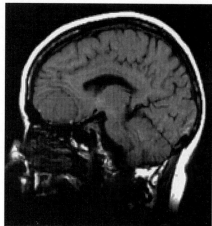
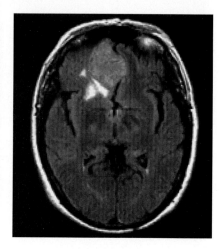

FIG. 37.1A   **FIG. 37.1B**   **FIG. 37.1C**

CLINICAL HISTORY

A 68-year-old woman with visual disturbances and headaches.

FINDINGS

A lobulated homogeneously enhancing mass is seen within the right frontal region. The mass has a broad base to both the falx and the cribriform plate. It is isointense to gray matter on T1-weighted images (Fig. 37.1A and B). The mass extends across the midline, deviating the falx. There is adjacent vasogenic edema within the right frontal lobe (Fig. 37.1C) on the FLAIR image. *Submitted by R.B. Muthyala, M.D., University of California, Irvine Medical Center, Orange, California, and William G. Bradley, M.D., Ph.D., F.A.C.R., Senior Editor, Long Beach Memorial Medical Center, Long Beach, California.*

DIAGNOSIS

Hemangiopericytoma.

DISCUSSION

Hemangiopericytoma is an uncommon soft tissue tumor, with 15% to 20% occurring in the head and neck and more than 50% of these occurring in the sinunasal tract (paranasal sinus and nasal cavity). Clinically, patients present with nasal obstruction and epistaxis. Hemangiopericytomas are believed to arise from spindle cells that surround blood vessels. They are highly vascular tumors. Roughly 10% have distant metastasis to the lung, with lymph node metastases being rare. They are considered radioresistant, with an approximately 60% recurrence rate if inadequately treated surgically.

On MRI, hemangiopericytomas are low to intermediate signal on T1-weighted images, bright on T2-weighted images, and generally show homogenous enhancement with gadolinium. They have a tendency to expand and remodel bone. Meningioma should be included in the differential diagnosis.

SUGGESTED READING

Compagno J. Hemangiopericytoma-like intranasal tumor. *Am J Clin Pathol* 1976;66:672.
Orrison WW. *Neuroimaging*. Philadelphia: WB Saunders, 1998.

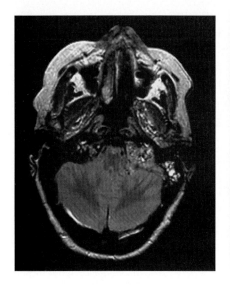

FIG. 38.1A

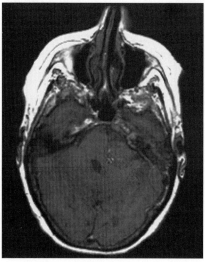

FIG. 38.1B

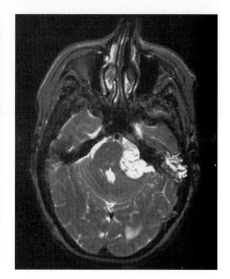

FIG. 38.1C

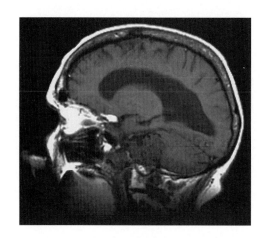

FIG. 38.1D

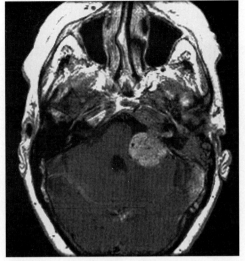
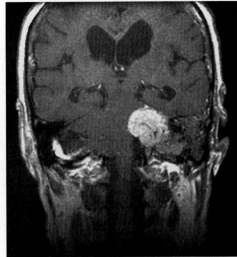

FIG. 38.1E   FIG. 38.1F

CLINICAL HISTORY

An 80-year-old woman with complaints of pulsatile tinnitus and difficulty hearing.

FINDINGS

There is a mass in the left cerebellopontine angle (Fig. 38.1A). On the T1-weighted image, the mass appears isointense to brain tissue (Fig. 38.1B). On the sagittal image, flow voids are noted, giving it a "salt and pepper" appearance (Fig. 38.1D). The T2-weighted axial image demonstrates hyperintensity of the mass (Fig. 38.1C). Postgadolinium coronal T1-weighted images show homogenous enhancement (Fig. 38.1E and F). *Submitted by R.B. Muthyala, M.D., University of California, Orange, California, and William G. Bradley, M.D., Ph.D., F.A.C.R., Senior Editor, Long Beach Memorial Medical Center, Long Beach, California.*

DIAGNOSIS

Glomus jugulare tumor.

DISCUSSION

Glomus jugulare, along with glomus tympanicum, is a benign tumor that arises from glomus bodies (paraganglioma tissue), which are located in the middle ear. Generally, they present with ringing in the ear and occur frequently in middle-aged woman. Glomus jugulare typically arises from the the auricular branches of the vagus nerve.

Radiographically on CT scan, they present as a soft tissue mass that erodes the jugular foramen. On MRI, multiple flow voids within the tumor give it a "salt and pepper" appearance. It is generally a homogenously enhancing, well-demarcated round or oval tumor. Paragangliomatosis is a hereditary condition associated with multiple glomus tumors and occurs in approximately 15% of patients with glomus tumor.

The differential diagnosis includes any mass in the jugular foramen. Included are schwannomas, enlarged jugular bulb (normal variant), metastasis, and meningiomas.

SUGGESTED READING

Grossman D. *Neuroradiology, the requisites.* St. Louis: Mosby–Year Book, 1994.
Orrison WW. *Neuroimaging.* Philadelphia: WB Saunders, 1998.

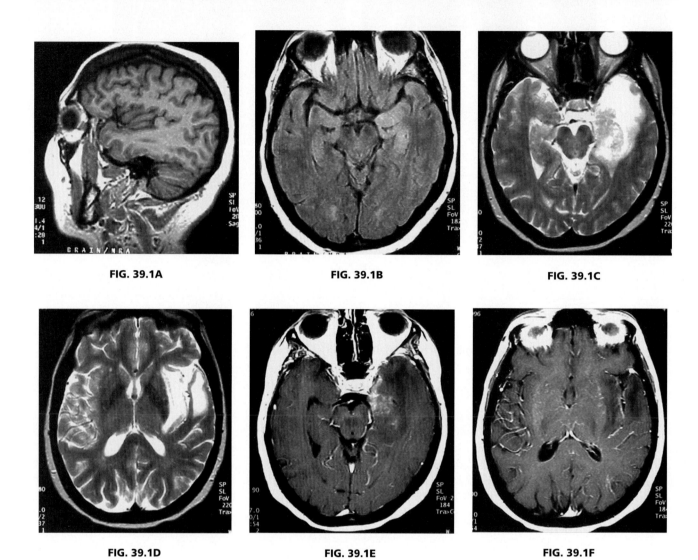

FIG. 39.1A

FIG. 39.1B

FIG. 39.1C

FIG. 39.1D

FIG. 39.1E

FIG. 39.1F

CLINICAL HISTORY

A 60-year-old woman with recent onset of confusion.

FINDINGS

Initially on admission, a sagittal noncontrast T1-weighted image (Fig. 39.1A) showed subtle thickening of the cortex within the medial left temporal lobe. Axial fluid-attenuated inversion-recovery (FLAIR) acquisition (Fig. 39.1B) demonstrated subtle gyriform high signal within the medial left temporal lobe in the region of the uncus. Additionally, there is swelling and medial displacement of the uncus.

The patient's symptomatology progressed and follow-up imaging was acquired 10 days later. Axial fast spin echo T2-weighted acquisition (Fig. 39.1C and D) is now markedly abnormal. There is diffuse abnormal high signal involving the cortex and subcortical white matter of the anterior and medial left temporal lobe, as well as extension of signal abnormality into the left insular cortex and perisylvian region. The right perisylvian region is also involved. The postcontrast axial T1-weighted acquisition (Fig. 39.1E and F) shows poorly defined cortical enhancement.

DIAGNOSIS

Herpes encephalitis.

DISCUSSION

Encephalitis is a diffuse, nonfocal inflammatory disease of the brain parenchyma. The etiology is usually viral, including nonepidemic (herpes simplex virus [HSV] types 1 and 2) and epidemic forms (Eastern, Western, and Venezuelan equine encephalitis). Slow-virus encephalitides include Creutzfeldt-Jakob disease and subacute sclerosing panencephalitis. Encephalitis in an immunocompromised host is usually caused by the human immunodeficiency virus itself, cytomegalovirus, and/or the papovavirus. Nonviral causes of encephalitis include *Toxoplasma gondii*, fungi, and *Listeria monocytogenes*.

The most common viral encephalitis in the United States and Europe is herpes simplex encephalitis (HSE). Herpes simplex type 2 (genital herpesvirus) is the cause of neonatal HSE, where the virus is contracted in the birth canal during a vaginal delivery. Herpes simplex type 1 (oral herpesvirus) is the cause of HSE in older infants, children, and adults (as seen in this case). During an oral herpes infection, the virus extends back to the gasserian ganglion. HSE is usually the result of activation of a latent infection in the gasserian ganglion; an encephalitis results from retrograde extension of the virus from the trigeminal ganglion into the brain.

HSE 1 occurs in both children and adults, and approximately one third of patients are less than 20 years of age. Patients typically develop a rapid change in mental status, seizures, fever, and headache. Early diagnosis is essential, as mortality rates for HSE are between 50% and 70%, with significant morbidity in surviving patients, whereas early therapy can be effective.

Pathologically, HSE is a fulminant hemorrhagic, necrotizing meningoencephalitis. The virus has a predilection for the limbic system, including the temporal lobes, cingulate gyri, and subfrontal region. Early in the course of the disease, CT is often normal. Low-density lesions may be seen in the temporal lobes with mild mass effect. Hemorrhage is characteristic of HSE but is not seen until the late stages of the disease on CT. Patchy ill-defined or gyriform enhancement may be seen following contrast. Early HSE is better detected with MRI. The early findings include thickened, edematous gyri on T1-weighted images. High signal is seen within the cortex and subcortical white matter of the temporal lobes and/or cingulate gyrus on T2-weighted images. Signal abnormality may extend into the insular cortex, usually sparing the putamen. FLAIR images have been shown to be more sensitive in the detection of subtle signal abnormalities seen in early disease. Enhancement and hemorrhage are unusual in the early stages of disease. The characteristic petechial hemorrhage associated with HSE is best seen on T1-weighted acquisition (more sensitive than CT). Follow-up scans (1 to 2 weeks after symptom onset) will demonstrate marked progression of disease, with extension of signal abnormality to involve the contralateral temporal lobe, cingulate gyrus, and insular cortex (as illustrated in this case). Hemorrhage and contrast enhancement may be more apparent.

Differential diagnosis is primarily low-grade glioma or infarct. Involvement of both temporal lobes and acute onset of symptoms would favor HSE over glioma. Cortical infarct should follow a vascular distribution. (White matter involvement is present acutely with HSE and develops later in infarcts.)

SUGGESTED READING

Demaerel P, Wilms G, Robberecht W, et al. MRI of herpes simplex encephalitis. *Neuroradiology* 1992;34(6):490–493.

Jacoby JH, diMarcangelo MT, Kramer ED. Imaging of herpes simplex encephalitis. *N Engl J Med* 1993;90(8):612–614.

Kato T, Ishii C, Furusho J, et al. Early diagnosis of herpes encephalopathy using fluid attenuated inversion recovery pulse sequences. *Pediatr Neurol* 1998;19(1):58–61.

Osborn AG. Infection, white matter abnormalities, and degenerative diseases. In: *Diagnostic neuroradiology*, 1st ed. St. Louis: Mosby, 1994:694–696.

White ML, Edwards-Brown MK. Fluid attenuated inversion recovery MRI in herpes encephalitis. *JCAT* 1995;19(3):501–502.

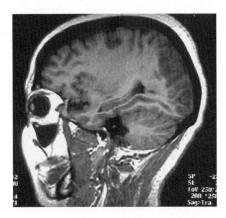

FIG. 40.1A

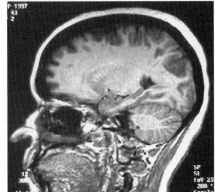

FIG. 40.1B

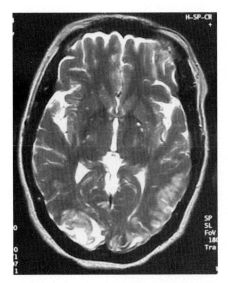

FIG. 40.1C

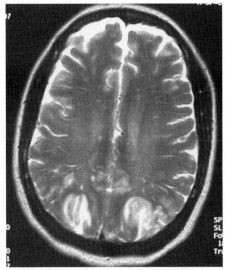

FIG. 40.1D

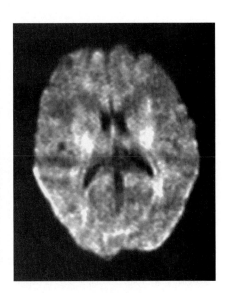

FIG. 40.1E

CLINICAL HISTORY

A 53-year-old woman with severe headache and blurred vision.

FINDINGS

Parasagittal T1-weighted acquisitions (Fig. 40.1A and B) demonstrate gyral low signal with thickening of the cortex involving the parietal and occipital lobes bilaterally. Axial fast spin echo T2-weighted acquisition (Fig. 40.1C and D) shows abnormal high signal involving the cortex and subcortical white matter in a similar distribution.

There is effacement of the overlying cortical sulci. There is no abnormal high signal on the T1-weighted acquisition to suggest hemorrhage. The dural venous sinus is patent.

Axial diffusion-weighted image (Fig. 40.1E) shows no signal abnormality to suggest acute ischemia.

DIAGNOSIS

Acute hypertensive encephalopathy.

DISCUSSION

Hypertensive encephalopathy is a syndrome characterized by reversible signal abnormality in the posterior regions of the brain in association with headache, mental status change, seizure, or visual disturbance. The most common etiologies include malignant hypertension, toxemia of pregnancy, immunosuppressive therapy (cyclosporin A toxicity) and chemotherapy (cisplatin and 5-fluorouracil). Uremic encephalopathy (related to chronic renal insufficiency, glomerulonephritis, hemolytic-uremic syndrome, or thrombotic thrombocytopenic purpura) can present with similar findings. In particular, erythropoietin (often used in chronic renal failure patients) has been found to be a causative agent in hypertensive posterior leukoencephalopathy syndromes. The syndrome is typically associated with acute hypertension, although patients may have little or no elevation of blood pressure. "Reversible posterior leukoencephalopathy syndrome" (RPLS) is a new, more inclusive term, that is being used to describe the characteristic clinical and radiographic findings of this entity, given the variable clinical settings discussed previously. Reversible occipitoparietal encephalopathy has more recently been suggested because of the involvement of both gray and white matter.

The classic imaging findings are bilateral, symmetric confluent regions of high signal on proton density–weighted, T2-weighted, and fluid-attenuated inversion-recovery images, involving the subcortical white matter of the parietal and occipital lobes with or without involvement of the overlying cortex. There is variable enhancement.

Another characteristic finding is edema within the basal ganglia, brainstem, and cerebellar hemispheres, characterized by swelling on T1-weighted images and hyperintense signal on T2-weighted images. Petechial hemorrhage in the affected areas is a distinguishing feature in RPLS and is seen as tiny foci of low signal on T2-weighted and gradient echo images. This finding is helpful in distinguishing nonspecific white matter disease from an acute or prior episode of hypertensive encephalopathy.

The pathophysiology of RPLS is ascribed to acute hypertension, which exceeds the brain's autoregulatory mechanism to preserve constant perfusion. The result is massive vasodilation of the cerebral arterioles, interruption of the blood–brain barrier, and extravasation of protein and fluid. Multifocal regions of interstitial edema ensue. The brain parenchyma supplied by the posterior circulation (vertebrobasilar system) is thought to be more affected because of a lesser degree of sympathetic innervation (support for the circulatory autoregulation mechanism) as compared with brain parenchyma supplied by the anterior circulation (internal cerebral arteries). The contention that hypertensive encephalopathy (or RPLS) is a reversible vasogenic edema, as opposed to a cytotoxic edema related to ischemia and/or infarction, is supported by the lack of signal abnormality on diffusion-weighted imaging (seen in this case). Diffusion-weighted imaging can therefore be instrumental in the diagnosis of RPLS.

Most cases will show reversal of clinical and imaging findings following normalization of blood pressure.

SUGGESTED READING

Hinchey J, Chaves C, Appignami B. A reversible posterior leukoencephalopathy syndrome. *N Engl J Med* 1996;22;334(8):494–500.

Ito Y, Arahata Y, Goto Y, et al. Cisplatin neurotoxicity presenting as reversible posterior leukoencephalopathy syndrome. *AJNR* 1998;19(3):415–417.

Pavlakis SG, Frank Y, Chusid R. Hypertensive encephalopathy/reversible occipitoparietal encephalopathy or reversible posterior leukoencephalopathy syndrome: three names for an old syndrome. *J Child Neurol* 1999;14(5):277–281.

Port JD, Beauchamp NJ Jr. Reversible intracranial pathologic entities mediated by vascular autoregulatory dysfunction. *Radiographics* 1998;18(2):353–367.

Schwartz RB, Bravo SM, Klufas RT, et al. Cyclosporine neurotoxicity and its relationship to hypertensive encephalopathy: CT and MR findings in 16 cases. *AJR* 1995;165(3):627–631.

Schwartz RB, Mulkern RV, Gudbjartsson H. Diffusion-weighted MR imaging in hypertensive encephalopathy: clues to the pathogenesis. *AJNR* 1998;19(5):859–862.

Weingarten K, Barbut D, Filippi C, et al. Acute hypertensive encephalopathy: findings on spin echo and gradient echo MR imaging. *AJR* 1994;162(3):665–670.

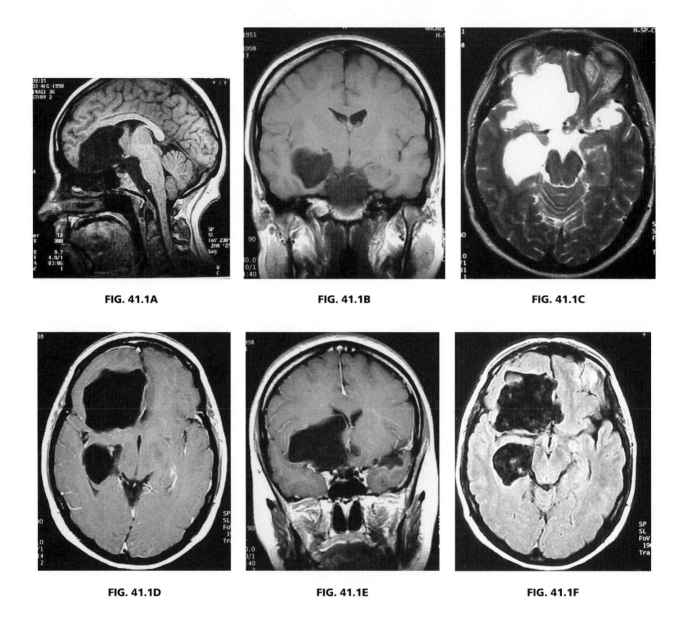

FIG. 41.1A **FIG. 41.1B** **FIG. 41.1C**

FIG. 41.1D **FIG. 41.1E** **FIG. 41.1F**

CLINICAL HISTORY

A 47-year-old woman with headache and cranial nerve palsy.

FINDINGS

Sagittal and coronal noncontrast T1-weighted acquisition (Fig. 41.1A and B) demonstrates a large, extraaxial well-defined hypointense mass within the subfrontal region, extending into the prepontine cistern with mass effect and posterior displacement of the thalami and brainstem, as well as superior displacement of the corpus callosum. The mass is slightly hyperintense to cerebrospinal fluid (CSF) on T1-weighted images and hypointense to CSF on the T2-weighted images (Fig. 41.1C). There is shift of the midline structures toward the left as well mass effect upon the right cerebral peduncle and frontal horn of the right lateral ventricle. Postcontrast image (Fig. 41.1D and E) shows no abnormal enhancement. There is subtle peripheral hyperintense signal suggestive of edema.

DIAGNOSIS

Epidermoid tumor.

DISCUSSION

Epidermoid tumors or cysts are slow-growing congenital inclusions, which are derived from tissues of epidermal origin. They are thought to result from the inclusion of epithelium during neural tube closure in the third to fifth week of embryogenesis (or rarely to result from traumatic or iatrogenic implantation of epidermal elements). They are composed of a wall of simple stratified squamous epithelium with a central collection of desquamative waxy keratin products. Epidermoids represent approximately 0.5% to 1.5% of all intracranial neoplasms. They are usually diagnosed later in life (second to fourth decade) because of their slow growth and limited symptomatology. The most common presenting complaints are seizure and headache in supratentorial lesions and cranial nerve dysfunction or vertigo in those below the tentorium. These tumors are extraaxial in location and occur most commonly within the cerebellopontine angle and parasellar regions. Other less common locations include the rhomboid fossa (ventral to the brainstem), ventricles and choroidal fissures, and subfrontal and interhemispheric regions. Fourth ventricular epidermoid tumors (see Case 23) account for about 16% of epidermoid tumors. Epidermoid tumors are typically located laterally (as opposed to the midline location of dermoid tumors). They grow locally and tend to insinuate themselves into the subarachnoid cisterns and sulci.

On CT, epidermoid tumors are lobulated extraaxial masses, which exhibit low density, similar to that of CSF. They may be slightly more dense than CSF and are rarely hyperdense. There may be internal tumor matrix. Enhancement is typically not seen. On MRI, epidermoid tumors are characteristically equal to or slightly higher in signal than CSF on all pulse sequences. The FLAIR acquisition is one of the most useful sequences in the diagnosis of epidermoid cyst, as they are almost always hyperintense to CSF on this sequence. The importance of evaluating the signal of the mass, as compared with CSF, is to differentiate epidermoid tumors from simple arachnoid cysts, which will follow CSF signal on all pulse sequences. MRI will often demonstrate internal architecture within epidermoid tumors, another distinguishing feature from arachnoid cyst. Diffusion-weighted imaging is the latest and most promising tool we have in the distinction of these entities. Using the differences in diffusion characteristics between the freely mobile protons within arachnoid cysts and the limited motion within the solid or semisolid matrix of epidermoid cysts, the distinction can be easily made. Epidermoid tumors demonstrate limited diffusion and appear bright on diffusion-weighted images while arachnoid cysts will follow CSF signal and appear dark. Magnetic resonance spectroscopy may also be helpful in the differentiation of these entities. Studies have shown the presence of a lactate peak in epidermoid cysts, whereas arachnoid cysts have minimal lactate on magnetic resonance spectroscopy.

SUGGESTED READING

Aprile I, Iariza F, Lavaroni A, et al. Analysis of cystic intracranial lesions performed with fluid-attenuated inversion recovery MR imaging. *AJNR* 1999;20(7):1,259–1,267.

Ikushima I, Korogi Y, Hirai T, et al. MR of epidermoids with a variety of pulse sequences. *AJNR* 1997;18(7):1,359–1,363.

Ishikawa M, Kikuchi H, Asato R. MR imaging of the intracranial epidermoid. *Acta Neurochir (Wien)* 1989;101(3-4):108–111.

Kallmes DF, Provenzale JM, Cloft HJ. Typical and atypical MR imaging features of intracranial epidermoid tumors. *AJR* 1997;169(3):883–887.

Panagopoulos KP, el-Azouzim, Chisholm HL, et al. Intracranial epidermoids. A continuing diagnostic challenge. *Arch Neurol* 1990;47(7):813–816.

Poptani H, Gupta RK, Jain VK. Cystic intracranial mass lesions: possible role of in vivo MR spectroscopy in its differential diagnosis. *Magn Reson Imaging* 1995;13(7):1,019–1,029.

Tsuruda JS, Chew WM, Moseley ME, et al. Diffusion-weighted MR imaging of the brain: value of differentiating between extraaxial cysts and epidermoid tumors. *AJR* 1990;155(5):1,059–1,065.

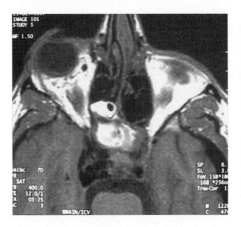

FIG. 42.1A

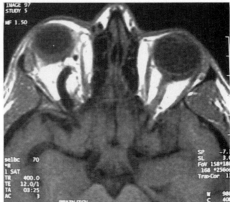

FIG. 42.1B

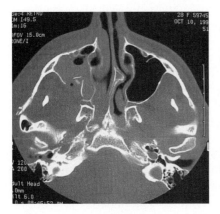

FIG. 42.1C

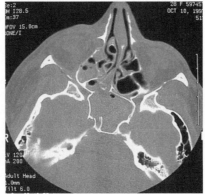

FIG. 42.1D

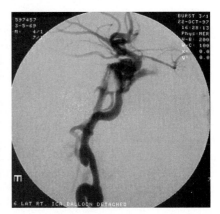

FIG. 42.1E

CLINICAL HISTORY

A 28-year-old woman with history of trauma.

FINDINGS

Axial T1-weighted acquisition (Fig. 42.1A) demonstrates prominent vessels in the region of the right cavernous sinus. Note convex lateral margin to the right cavernous sinus. More superiorly (Fig. 42.1B), there is marked enlargement of the superior ophthalmic vein. There is proptosis of the right globe.

DIAGNOSIS

Posttraumatic carotid-cavernous fistula.

DISCUSSION

Despite missing traumatic skull fractures given the absence of high-resolution imaging of bone, MRI is quite useful in detecting the parenchymal and vascular sequelae of head trauma. In this case, the prominence of the cavernous sinus and serpentine channels in the region of the cavernous sinus suggest the presence of a vascular shunt. The enlargement of the superior thalamic vein and proptosis are further corroborating evidence. Clinically, the patient exhibited proptosis and slight ecchymosis of the lower eyelid. In the setting of known head trauma, a tear of the carotid artery with communication to the cavernous sinus at the skull base is the most likely explanation for this syndrome. CT scanning verifies the traumatic fracture of the skull base (Fig. 42.1C and D).

Any skull base fracture that extends to the sphenoid bone should be investigated further with either magnetic resonance or conventional angiography to verify integrity of the carotid artery or demonstrate any disruption such as pseudoaneurysm or traumatic carotid-cavernous fistula. The fistulae can be treated with endovascular technique. Such fistulae may constitute a neurosurgical/ophthalmologic emergency if vision deteriorates suddenly due to elevation of superior ophthalmic venous pressure from the fistulae's flow or thrombosis of the vein (which can occur in these cases).

Selected frame from lateral view right carotid angiogram (Fig. 42.1E) shows an abnormal communication between the cavernous internal carotid artery and cavernous sinus with early filling of the inferior petrosal sinus confirming the presence of a traumatic carotid-cavernous fistula. Also note dissection of the high cervical carotid artery.

SUGGESTED READING

Barrow DL, Spector RD, Braun IF, et al. Classification and treatment of spontaneous carotid cavernous sinus fistulas. *J Neurosurg* 1985;62:248–256.

Guo WY, Pan DHC, Wu HM, et al. Radiosurgery as a treatment alternative for dural arteriovenous fistulas of the cavernous sinus. *AJNR* 1998;19:1,081–1,087.

Vinuela F, Fox A, Debrun GM, et al. Spontaneous carotid fistula: clinical, radiological, and therapeutic considerations. *J Neurosurg* 1984;60:976–984.

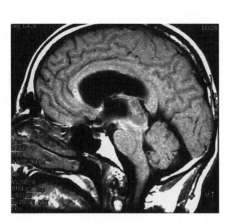

FIG. 43.1A

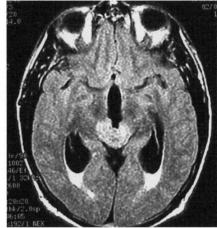

FIG. 43.1B

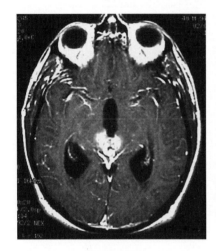

FIG. 43.1C

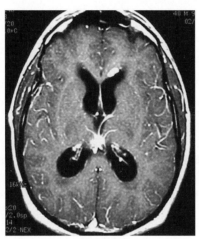

FIG. 43.1D

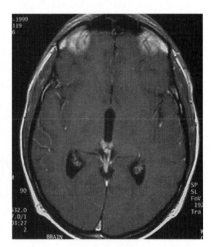

FIG. 43.1E

CLINICAL HISTORY

A 40-year-old man with history of Parinaud syndrome.

FINDINGS

Sagittal T1-weighted acquisition (Fig. 43.1A) demonstrates a large multilobulated isointense mass in the region of the pineal gland. There is mass effect upon the dorsal aspect of the midbrain with obstruction of the cerebral aqueduct. Note dilation of the lateral and third ventricles. Axial fluid-attenuated inversion-recovery acquisition (Fig. 43.1B) shows a hyperintense mass along the posterior aspect of the third ventricle in the expected location of the pineal gland. There is periventricular high signal surrounding the atria of the lateral ventricles, due to the accumulation of cerebrospinal fluid (CSF) related to the obstructive hydrocephalus. Postcontrast T1-weighted acquisition (Fig. 43.1C) shows heterogenous enhancement of the mass. Note nodules of enhancement along the ependyma of the frontal horns of the lateral ventricles (Fig. 43.1D).

DIAGNOSIS

Germinoma with transependymal spread of tumor.

DISCUSSION

Germinomas are tumors of germ cell origin that account for approximately 0.5% to 2.0% of primary intracranial tumors. Their histology is similar to that of ovarian dysgerminoma and testicular seminoma. These tumors account for 40% of pineal region masses. Other less common pineal germ cell tumors include choriocarcinoma, embryonal cell carcinoma, endodermal sinus tumor, and teratoma. Intracranial germ cell tumors usually occur in the midline, most commonly in the pineal region followed by the suprasellar region and fourth ventricle. Germ cell tumors involving the basal ganglia and thalamus are less common. Occasionally, there are metachronous pineal and suprasellar germinomas.

Germinomas usually present between the ages of 5 and 25. There is a male predominance in pineal tumors with no sex predilection in suprasellar lesions. Presenting symptoms include paresis of upward gaze (Parinaud syndrome), hydrocephalus, precocious puberty, and diabetes insipidus, depending on tumor location.

The classic appearance on CT is a hyperdense mass on unenhanced scans that demonstrates intense enhancement following contrast. It is said that pineal germinomas often calcify, but there is debate as to whether it is calcification of the tumor itself or the normally calcified pineal gland engulfed by tumor. The normal pineal gland is calcified in 10% of patients 8 to 14 years old and 40% of patients by 20 years of age.

Pineal germinomas are well-circumscribed lesions that are inseparable from the gland itself. Invasion of adjacent brain parenchyma and CSF seeding are common associated findings. Suprasellar germinomas, however, tend to be very infiltrative and have a propensity to spread throughout the subarachnoid space, coating the basal cisterns, optic nerves/chiasm, and ventricular walls with tumor. "Drop metastases" into the spinal canal can occur with germinomas in any location (8% to 18% of cases).

On MRI, germinomas have intermediate signal intensity on T1-weighted images and isointense to hypointense signal on T2-weighted images because of the tumor cells' high nuclear-to-cytoplasm ratio. Germinomas are usually homogeneous tumors, however, intratumoral hemorrhage is common. Cystic change is variable. Germinomas are uniquely sensitive to radiation therapy and have good survival rates even in the face of diffuse metastases; 5-year survival rates are from 80% to 90%.

One month later, following radiation therapy (2,000 Gy) in this patient, a follow-up scan was acquired. Postcontrast T1-weighted image (Fig. 43.1E) shows marked response of the tumor to radiation therapy. The nodules of enhancement within the frontal horns are no longer identified. There is significant improvement of the hydrocephalus, compared with the findings in the previous study.

The primary differential diagnosis for pineal germinoma includes other germ cell tumors and pineal cell tumors (pineoblastoma and pineocytoma). The less common germ cell tumors (such as teratoma, choriocarcinoma, embryonal cell carcinoma, and endodermal sinus tumor) have variable signal on MRI and often cannot be distinguished from germinoma based on imaging alone. Serum markers can be helpful in differentiating these tumors. Teratomas are characteristically very heterogeneous in signal due to cystic change, fat, calcification, and hemorrhage. There is variable enhancement.

Pineoblastomas occur in children and are classified as a primitive neuroectodermal tumor histologically. They are very aggressive and disseminate throughout the subarachnoid space early in their course. The prognosis is poor. Pineocytoma occurs in middle-aged to older adults. These are well-defined tumors that typically do not infiltrate brain or CSF pathways. Both pineoblastomas and pineocytomas are solid, lobulated pineal region masses that enhance on CT and MRI. Because of their dense cellularity, pineoblastomas (like germinomas) are usually isointense to hypointense to gray matter on T2-weighted images. Pineocytoma is relatively higher in signal on long TE images. Both lesions can calcify, although this is more common with pineocytoma.

Other pineal region masses to consider in the differential diagnoses include glioma, meningioma, choroid plexus papilloma, metastases, vascular lesions, and nonneoplastic masses such as pineal cyst, arachnoid cyst, lipoma, and epidermoid and dermoid cyst.

SUGGESTED READING

Choi JU, Kim DS, Chung SS, et al. Treatment of germ cell tumors in the pineal region. *Child Nerv Syst* 1998;14:41–48.

Fujimaki T, Matsutani M, Funada N, et al. CT and MRI features of intracranial germ cell tumors. *J Neurooncol* 1994;19(3):217–226.

Higano S, Takahashi S, Ishi K, et al. Germinoma originating in the basal ganglia and thalamus: CT and MRI evaluation. *AJNR* 1994;15(8):1,435–1,441.

Maroldo TV, Barkovich AJ. Pediatric brain tumors. *Semin Ultrasound Comput Tomogr Magn Reson* 1992;13:412–448.

Sumida M, Uozumi T, Kiya K, et al. MRI of intracranial germ cell tumors. *Neuroradiology* 1995;37(1):32–37.

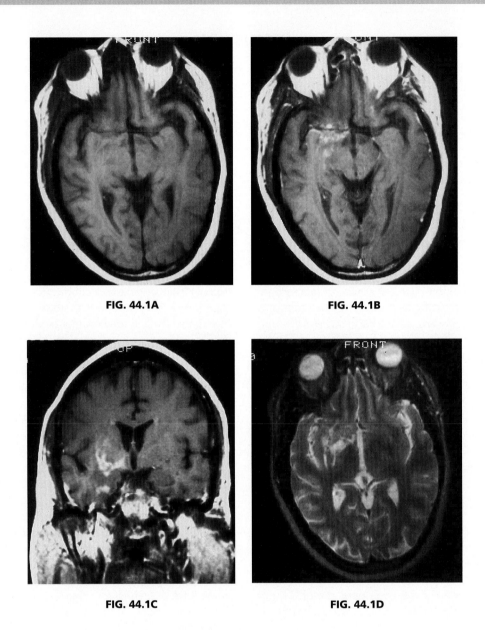

FIG. 44.1A

FIG. 44.1B

FIG. 44.1C

FIG. 44.1D

CLINICAL HISTORY

A 44-year-old African American woman presenting with severe headaches.

FINDINGS

Abnormal enhancement is noted in the cistern of the M_1 segment of the right middle cerebral artery and in the right perimesenphalic cistern (Fig. 44.1A and B). On postcontrast coronal views, this enhancement is noted to extend up from the cistern of the middle cerebral artery along the lenticulostriate arteries into the basal ganglia (Fig. 44.1C). High signal intensity is noted in this region on T2-weighted images (Fig. 44.1D). *Submitted by William G. Bradley, M.D., Ph.D., F.A.C.R., Senior Editor, Long Beach Memorial Medical Center, Long Beach, California.*

DIAGNOSIS

Sarcoidosis.

DISCUSSION

Sarcoidosis is an inflammatory systemic disease of uncertain etiology. In the brain, it has a propensity for the leptomeninges and the pituitary stalk. It is characterized by leptomeningeal enhancement, in this case extending into the Virchow-Robin spaces surrounding the lenticulostriate arteries arising from the M_1 segment of the middle cerebral artery. It is more common in African Americans.

Pathologically, sarcoidosis is similar to tuberculosis in that both are granulomatosis diseases. They are distinguished by the fact that sarcoid granulomas do not caseate, whereas tuberculosis granulomas do. The diagnosis is confirmed by a skin test called the "Kveim test."

SUGGESTED READING

Christoforidis GA, Spickler EM, Recio MV, et al. MR of CNS sarcoidosis: correlation of imaging features to clinical symptoms and response to treatment. *AJNR* 1999;20(4):655–669.

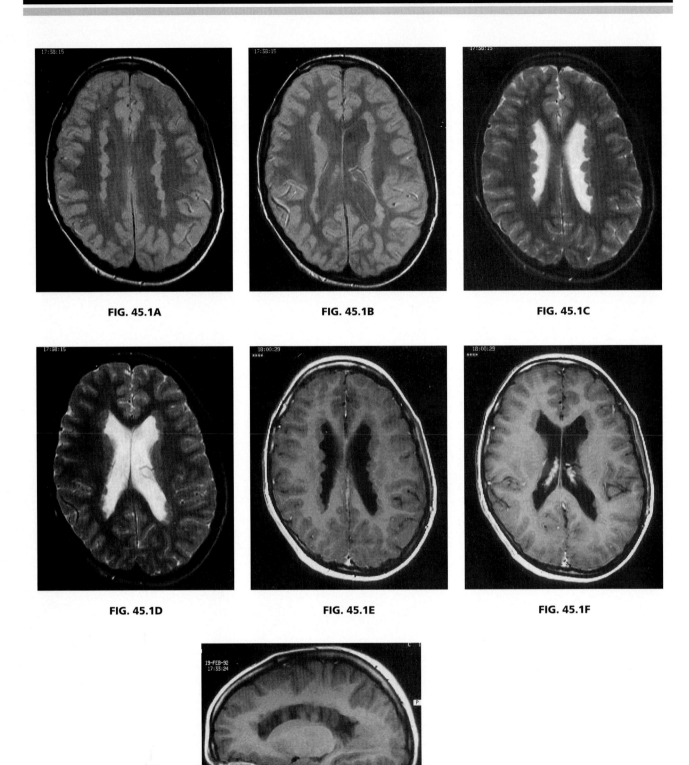

FIG. 45.1A

FIG. 45.1B

FIG. 45.1C

FIG. 45.1D

FIG. 45.1E

FIG. 45.1F

FIG. 45.1G

CLINICAL HISTORY

A 14-year-old girl with seizures.

FINDINGS

Multiple T1-weighted, proton density, and T2-weighted axial and sagittal images demonstrate nodules with the same intensity as gray matter along the lateral aspect of the lateral ventricles (Fig. 45.1A–G). *Submitted by William G. Bradley, M.D., Ph.D., F.A.C.R., Senior Editor, Long Beach Memorial Medical Center, Long Beach, California.*

DIAGNOSIS

Heterotopic gray matter.

DISCUSSION

Heterotopic gray matter is a failure of migration of neurons from the germinal matrix centrally to the cortex peripherally. Patients generally present with seizures or mental retardation. The nodules show no evidence of enhancement (Fig. 45.1E and F), as they are essentially normal gray matter.

The main element in the differential diagnosis is tuberous sclerosis with subependymal hamartomas. At this age, most of these tubers would have calcified were this tuberous sclerosis.

SUGGESTED READING

Zimmerman RA, Bilaniuk LT. Pediatric cerebral anomalies. In: Stark DD, Bradley WG, eds. *Magnetic resonance imaging,* 3rd ed. St. Louis: Mosby, 1999:1,403–1,425.

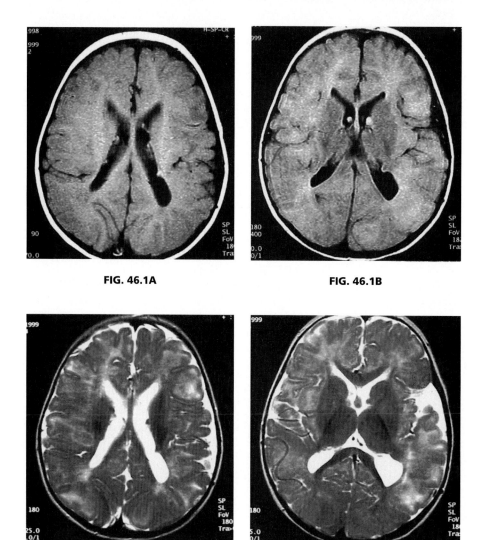

FIG. 46.1A

FIG. 46.1B

FIG. 46.1C

FIG. 46.1D

CLINICAL HISTORY

A 7-month-old girl with seizures.

FINDINGS

Axial T1-weighted acquisition (Fig. 46.1A and B) demonstrates multiple subependymal nodules within the lateral ventricles bilaterally, as well as nodules at the foramen of Monro. The nodules are hyperintense as compared with normal gray matter on the T1-weighted acquisition. Axial T2-weighted images (Fig. 46.1C and D) demonstrate hypointense nodules as compared with gray matter. The ventricles are normal in size. There are multiple patchy, poorly defined regions of high signal involving the cortex and subcortical white matter of both cerebral hemispheres.

DIAGNOSIS

Tuberous sclerosis.

DISCUSSION

Tuberous sclerosis (Bourneville disease) is an inherited, autosomal dominant disease. More than 50% of cases, however, arise via spontaneous mutation. The characteristic clinical triad is adenoma sebaceum, mental retardation, and seizures. All three occur together in only one third of cases. The prevalence of epilepsy in tuberous sclerosis is over 80%. The typical intracranial findings include periventricular subependymal nodules, cortical and subcortical tubers, white matter lesions, and subependymal giant cell astrocytomas. Heterotopias and ventriculomegaly can also be present. Other systemic manifestations include retinal hamartomas, shagreen patches, ungual fibromas, rhabdomyomas of the heart, angiomyolipomas of the kidney, pulmonary lymphangioleiomyomatosis, and cystic osseous lesions. The pathogenesis of the intracranial lesions is thought to be due to abnormal radial-glial migration of dysgenetic cells that have the potential to differentiate into astrocytes or neurons, resulting in focal hamartomatous lesions and/or migration anomalies.

Subependymal nodules are small lesions, which usually do not grow but progressively calcify with age. Most subependymal nodules are calcified by the age of 20. These lesions are more easily seen on CT because of their high density, which contrasts with surrounding low-density CSF. On MRI, their signal is variable. Often, there is a central core of high signal on T2-weighted images producing a "target" appearance. Occasionally on T1-weighted images, there will be central hyperintensity due to the paradoxical high signal that can occur with microscopic calcification. Subependymal nodules have variable patterns of enhancement. If there is enhancement on CT, it is considered diagnostic of conversion of the nodule into a giant cell astrocytoma. On MRI, subependymal nodules can enhance, and

only if the enhancing nodule is large, solitary, and in the region of the foramen of Monro should the possibility of giant cell astrocytoma be considered.

Multiple cortical tubers are diagnostic of tuberous sclerosis. Fifty percent of cortical hamartomas will calcify (often wedge shaped). Noncalcified tubers usually appear as low-density cortical/subcortical lesions on unenhanced CT. In older patients, noncalcified cortical tubers are high signal on T2-weighted acquisition and low signal on T1-weighted images. They often appear as large misshapen gyri. Only rarely do they show contrast enhancement.

White matter abnormality in tuberous sclerosis is better identified on MRI. These lesions appear as linear or curvilinear thin bands of high signal on T2-weighted images, which often connect subependymal nodules with cortical tubers. Wedge-shaped or tumefactive white matter lesions can also be found in tuberous sclerosis. Enhancement is variable.

In infants (less than 3 months of age), the signal intensity of the subependymal and parenchymal lesions is reversed. Lesions are high signal on T1-weighted images and low signal on T2-weighted acquisition. The conspicuity of white matter lesions is maintained in infants because of sparse myelination. Purely intracortical lesions are more difficult to identify. Cortical tubers in infants can be large and hyperattenuating on CT, simulating hemorrhagic infarcts or calcification.

Subependymal giant cell astrocytomas are benign, slow-growing tumors that occur in up to 15% of patients with tuberous sclerosis. They are typically large solitary high-signal lesions at the foramen of Monro on T2-weighted images. There is moderate enhancement and rarely calcification. The malignant potential is low and morbidity is related to ventricular obstruction.

SUGGESTED READING

Altman NR, Purser RK, Donovan Post MJ. Tuberous sclerosis: characteristics at CT and MRI imaging. *Radiology* 1988;167:527–532.

Barkovich AJ, Baron Y. Magnetic resonance imaging of tuberous sclerosis in neonates and young infants. *AJNR* 1999;20(5):907–916.

Kotagal P, Rothner AD. Epilepsy in the setting of neurocutaneous syndromes. *Epilepsia* 1993;34(Suppl 3):71–78.

Smirniotopoulos JG, Murphy FM. Central nervous system manifestations of the phakomatoses and other inherited syndromes. In: Atlas SW, ed. *Magnetic resonance imaging of the brain and spine,* 2nd ed. Philadelphia: Lippincott–Raven Publishers, 1996;786–790.

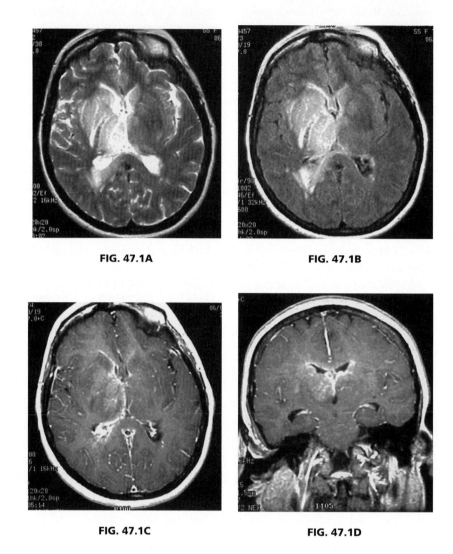

FIG. 47.1A   **FIG. 47.1B**

FIG. 47.1C   **FIG. 47.1D**

CLINICAL HISTORY

A 55-year-old woman with development of stupor in the past 24 hours. Four days prior to admission, the patient had dental work performed, and on the day of admission, she had developed vomiting followed by drowsiness.

FINDINGS

Axial fast spin echo T2-weighted acquisition and fluid-attenuated inversion-recovery images (Fig. 47.1A and B) demonstrate diffuse, poorly defined abnormal high signal involving the right basal ganglia, thalamus, and deep periventricular white matter adjacent to the atrium of the right lateral ventricle. Additionally, there is high signal within the left basal ganglia. The ventricles are normal in size. Following intravenous contrast (Fig. 47.1C), there is abnormal enhancement within the right basal ganglia as well as along the ependyma of the right and left lateral ventricle. Coronal postcontrast acquisition (Fig. 47.1D) shows no abnormal meningeal enhancement.

DIAGNOSIS

Cerebritis with associated ventriculitis.

DISCUSSION

Cerebritis is the earliest stage of brain infection. It often progresses to cerebral abscess in a predictable pattern (see Case 31). Pathologically, cerebritis is a localized yet poorly defined area of softened parenchyma with scattered necrosis, edema, vascular congestion, petechial hemorrhage, and inflammatory infiltrate. It can result from direct spread of infection from sinus or mastoid air cells, overlying meningitis, or from hematogenous spread from an extracranial site of infection. The specific organisms involved are quite variable, and often, more than one organism is involved. Cerebritis is usually bacterial (streptococcus or staphylococcus) but can be due to tuberculosis, fungi, or parasites.

T2-weighted images feature an ill-defined region of increased signal, which is indistinguishable from surrounding edema. T1-weighted images show an isointense to hypointense lesion with perifocal mass effect manifested as sulcal effacement and ipsilateral ventricular compression. There can be hyperintense foci if petechial hemorrhage is present. Contrast enhancement is minimal and inhomogeneous.

A focus of cerebritis progresses to abscess when the central necrotic zones become liquefied and a better defined capsule can be identified. When an abscess forms, an irregular ring-enhancing mass lesion is seen on postcontrast imaging (see Case 31).

Complications of cerebritis include ventriculitis (as seen in this case) and meningitis. The primary differential diagnosis for a parenchymal mass lesion with ventricular involvement is cerebritis/ventriculitis or glioma with subependymal spread of tumor.

SUGGESTED READING

Hansman Whiteman ML, Bowen BC, Donovan Post MJ, et al. Intracranial infection. In: Atlas SW, ed. *Magnetic resonance imaging of the brain and spine,* 2nd ed. Philadelphia: Lippincott–Raven Publishers, 1996:726–729.

Hatta H, Mochizuki H, Kuru Y, et al. Serial neuroradiological studies in focal cerebritis. *Neuroradiology* 1994;36(4):285–288.

Sze G, Zimmerman RD. The magnetic resonance imaging of infections and inflammatory diseases. *Radiol Clin North Am* 1988;26:839–859.

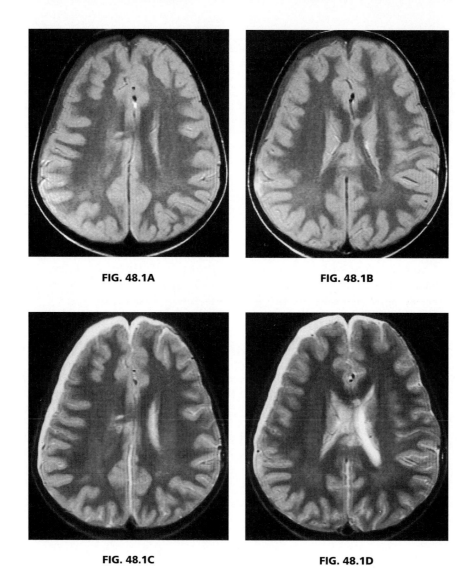

FIG. 48.1A

FIG. 48.1B

FIG. 48.1C

FIG. 48.1D

CLINICAL HISTORY

A 5-year-old boy following head trauma.

FINDINGS

Proton density–weighted (Fig. 48.1A and B) and T2-weighted (Fig. 48.1C and D) images in the axial plane through the lateral ventricles demonstrate high signal intensity areas in the corpus callosum. There is also an extraaxial fluid collection over the right frontal convexity, which has the same intensity as cerebrospinal fluid (CSF). *Submitted by William G. Bradley, M.D., Ph.D., F.A.C.R., Senior Editor, Long Beach Memorial Medical Center, Long Beach, California.*

DIAGNOSES

(i) Shear injury and (ii) subdural CSF collection due to an arachnoid rent (subdural hygroma).

DISCUSSION

Shear injury, also called "diffuse axonal injury," results from rotational forces applied to the brain during head trauma. It most commonly affects the gray-white junction, the corpus callosum (as in this case), the posterior limb of the internal capsule, and the posterolateral upper brainstem. Shear injury can be bland or hemorrhagic; only the latter is visible, as punctate high density on CT. Shear injury should be suspected when the Glasgow coma scale score remains depressed in the setting of normal intracranial pressure and an ostensibly normal CT scan. MRI is the preferred technique for making this diagnosis.

The term "subdural hygroma" has been used by some to mean a chronic subdural hematoma and by others to mean a CSF collection in the subdural space due to an arachnoid tear. (The CSF normally resides beneath the arachnoid membrane in the subarachnoid space.) When there is a rent in the arachnoid, a one-way ball-valve mechanism can lead to a CSF collection in the subdural space, as is shown here. The differentiation between a CSF collection and chronic hemorrhage is best made on proton density or fluid-attenuated inversion-recovery images, which are sensitive to small changes in T1 due to protein content, chronic subdural hematomas always appearing brighter than CSF.

SUGGESTED READING

Bradley WG. Brainstem: normal anatomy and pathology. In: Stark DD, Bradley WG, eds. *Magnetic resonance imaging*, 3rd ed. St. Louis: Mosby, 1999:1,187–1,208.
Gentry LR, Godersky JC, Thompson BH. Traumatic brainstem injury: MR imaging. *Radiology* 1989;171:177.

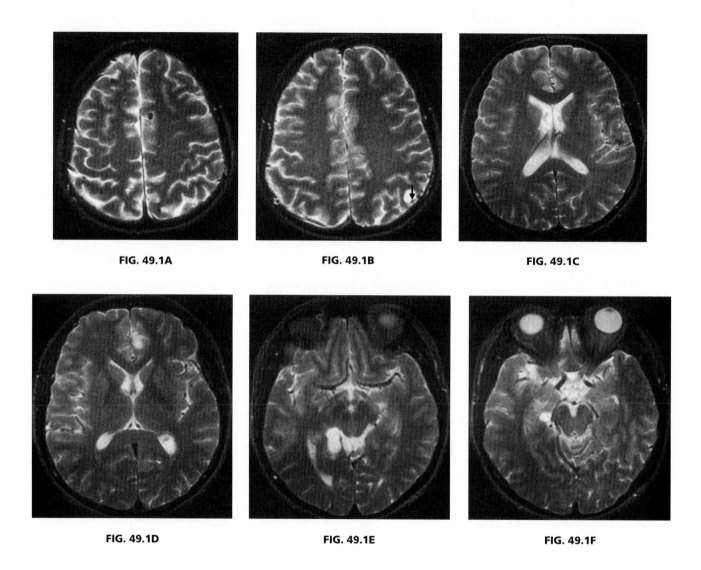

FIG. 49.1A   FIG. 49.1B   FIG. 49.1C

FIG. 49.1D   FIG. 49.1E   FIG. 49.1F

CLINICAL HISTORY

A 36-year-old Mexican man with seizures for the last 20 years.

FINDINGS

T2-weighted images through the supratentorial region demonstrate multiple areas of punctate low signal intensity (Fig. 49.1A and C) as well as focal areas of rounded high signal within the parenchyma (Fig. 49.1B) and subarachnoid space (Fig. 49.1D–F) without vasogenic edema. *Submitted by William G. Bradley, M.D., Ph.D., F.A.C.R., Senior Editor, Long Beach Memorial Medical Center, Long Beach, California.*

DIAGNOSIS

Cysticercosis.

DISCUSSION

Cysticercosis is by far the most common cause of seizures in Mexico. For this reason, in many parts of Mexico patients presenting with first-time seizures are treated with praziquantel, rather than studied by CT or MRI. Cysticercosis most commonly involves the brain, where it can appear as cystic lesions with a small scolex (Fig. 49B, *small arrow*). When the scolex dies, an inflammatory reaction results in vasogenic edema and enhancement (not shown in this case). Ultimately, the inflammatory reaction results in focal calcification, seen as low-intensity areas on MRI.

SUGGESTED READING

Martinez HR, Rangel-Guerra R, Elizondo G, et al. MR imaging in neurocysticercosis: study of 56 cases. *Am J Neuroradiol* 1989;10:1,011.

Teitelbaum GP, Otto RJ, Linn MCW, et al. MR imaging of neurocysticercosis. *Am J Neuroradiol* 1989;10:709.

Zee CS, Segall HD, Apuzzo MLJ. Intraventricular cysticercal cysts: further neuroradiologic observations and neurosurgical implications. *Am J Neuroradiol* 1984;5:727.

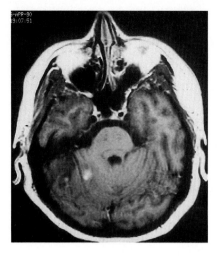

FIG. 50.1A

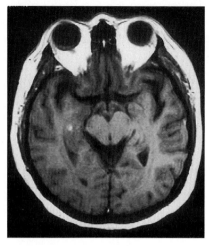

FIG. 50.1B

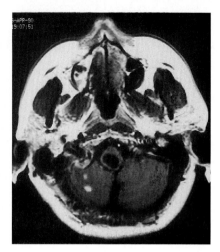

FIG. 50.1C

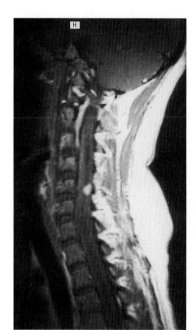

FIG. 50.1D

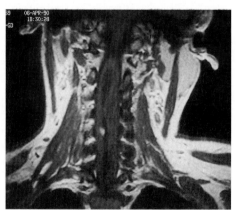

FIG. 50.1E

CLINICAL HISTORY

A 31-year-old woman with headaches, decreasing visual acuity, upper neck pain, and numbness in the arms.

FINDINGS

Enhanced T1-weighted axial images through the cerebellum oral temporal lobe demonstrate multiple enhancing nodules (Fig. 50.1A–C). The presence of a syrinx (Fig. 50.1C) prompted a cervical spine examination, which demonstrated an additional nodule (Fig. 50.1D and E). On ophthalmologic examination, bilateral retinal angiomas were detected. Patient also gave a history of three family members with von Hippel-Lindau (VHL) syndrome. *Submitted by William G. Bradley, M.D., Ph.D., F.A.C.R., Senior Editor, Long Beach Memorial Medical Center, Long Beach, California.*

DIAGNOSIS

Hemangioblastomas (VHL).

DISCUSSION

VHL is a disorder diagnosed on the basis of the constellation of imaging findings, rather than a defined chromosomal abnormality. Approximately one third of all patients with VHL have cerebellar hemangioblastomas and one third of patients with cerebellar hemangioblastomas have VHL. The combination of spinal and cerebellar hemangioblastomas is diagnostic of VHL. The combination of cerebellar hemangioblastomas with retinal angiomas is diagnostic of VHL. These patients also tend to get cystic lesions of the epididymis, pancreas, etc.

Whenever an enhancing cystic mass is noted in the cerebellum, the spine should also be scanned for similar lesions, and vice versa.

SUGGESTED READING

Hasso AN, Bell SA, Tadmor R. Intracranial vascular tumors. *Neuroimaging Clin N Am* 1994;4(4):449–480.

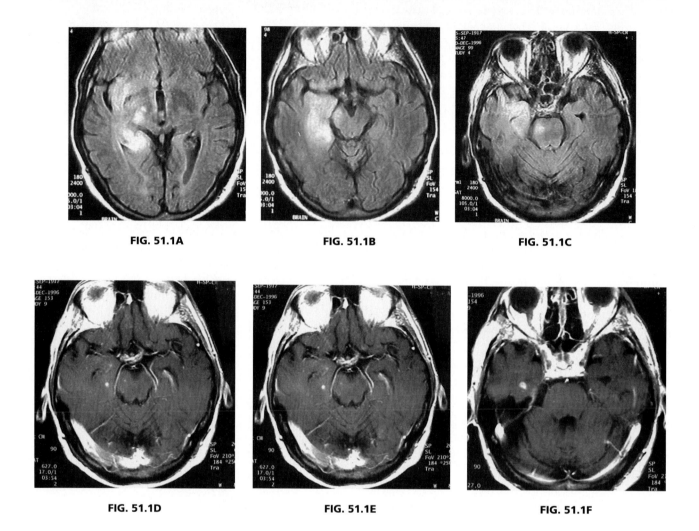

FIG. 51.1A   FIG. 51.1B   FIG. 51.1C

FIG. 51.1D   FIG. 51.1E   FIG. 51.1F

CLINICAL HISTORY

A 79-year-old man with memory difficulties.

FINDINGS

Axial fluid-attenuated inversion-recovery acquisition (Fig. 51.1A–C) demonstrates hyperintense signal within the medial right temporal lobe extending into the region of the insular cortex and right cerebral peduncle. There is also a focus of abnormal high signal within the right side of the pons.

Postcontrast acquisition (Fig. 51.1D–F) shows several small foci of enhancement within the right temporal lobe and brainstem. There is mild mass effect upon the temporal horn of the right lateral ventricle, as well as mild medial displacement of the uncus.

DIAGNOSIS

Gliomatosis cerebri (GC).

DISCUSSION

GC is a diffusely infiltrative glial neoplasm that primarily involves the cerebral hemispheres and brainstem. The cerebellum and spinal cord can also be affected. Whether GC is a distinct pathologic entity or an early form of anaplastic astrocytoma or glioblastoma multiforme with extraordinary infiltrative features remains a controversy.

GC is a rare entity that can occur at any age, although it commonly presents in the second to fourth decade of life. Clinically, personality and/or mental status changes are noted, which are mild relative to the extent of involvement as seen on imaging.

GC typically involves both white and gray matter, although the white matter disease predominates at imaging. There is characteristic enlargement of the involved cerebral/cerebellar hemisphere or brainstem with relative preservation of normal underlying anatomic architecture. Tumor can be more concentrated in certain parts of the brain; however, there are generally no focal mass lesions identifiable. Although any portion of the brain can be involved, GC has a predilection for the optic nerves and other compact white matter tracts. The corpus callosum, fornices, and cerebellar peduncles are frequently involved. Primary leptomeningeal gliomatosis can also occur.

Pathologically, there are infiltrative neoplastic astrocytes in different stages of differentiation arranged in a perineuronal and perivascular distribution. There is thickening of the white matter tracts with extensive demyelination in the involved areas.

MRI features include large, confluent, ill-defined regions of high signal on T2-weighted images primarily involving hemispheric white matter with or without involvement of the brainstem and overlying cortex. The corpus callosum is often involved. There is typically expansion of the involved white matter tracts. Cortical sulci are well preserved, but ventricles may be asymmetrically small. Poor delineation between gray and white matter is described as a characteristic finding in this condition. Imaging findings in GC can be indistinguishable from those of demyelinating disease and biopsy is often required to secure the diagnosis. GC typically does not enhance, although foci of enhancement can be seen late in the disease and with leptomeningeal involvement.

GC will often respond to steroids and/or radiation therapy in the short term, but the long-term prognosis is poor, with focal dedifferentiation to glioblastoma common.

SUGGESTED READING

Kim DG, Yang HJ, Park IA, et al. Gliomatosis cerebri: clinical features, treatment and prognosis. *Acta Neurochir (Wien)* 1998;140(8):755–762.

Keene DL, Jimenez C, Hsu E. MRI diagnosis of gliomatosis cerebri. *Pediatr Neurol* 1999;20(2):148–151.

Martinez-Mata AM, Martinez-Pardavila R, de Arriba-Villamor C, et al. Cerebral gliomatosis with development of multifocal glioblastoma. *Rev Neurol* 1999;28(8):781–783.

Ponce P, Alvarez-Santullano MV, Otermin E, et al. Gliomatosis cerebri: findings with computed tomography and magnetic resonance imaging. *Eur J Radiol* 1998;28(3):226–229.

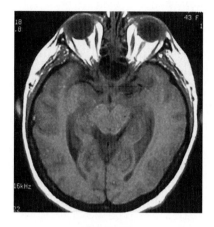

FIG. 52.1A

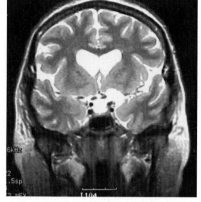

FIG. 52.1B

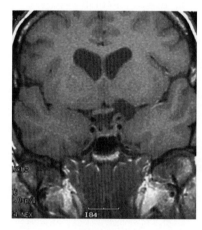

FIG. 52.1C

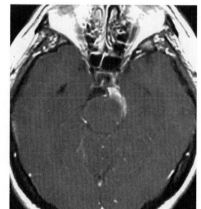

FIG. 52.1D

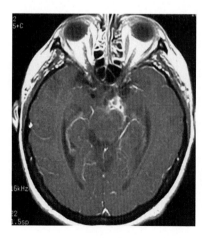

FIG. 52.1E

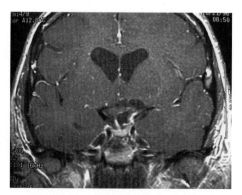

FIG. 52.1F

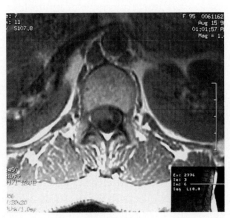

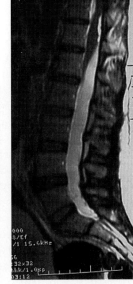

FIG. 52.1G   **FIG. 52.1H**

CLINICAL HISTORY

A 43-year-old woman with headaches and visual disturbance.

FINDINGS

Axail T1-weighted and coronal fast spin echo T2-weighted images (Fig. 52.1A and B) demonstrate a cystic lesion within the left parasellar region, which follows cerebrospinal fluid (CSF) signal on both pulse sequences. Targeted coronal T1-weighted images through the sella turcica (Fig. 52.1C) show mass effect upon the left thalamus, as well as rightward deviation of the infundibulum and optic chiasm. There is intermediate signal-enhancing material encasing the left middle cerebral artery within the suprasellar cistern. Note abnormal enhancement in the left suprasellar and prepontine cisterns (Fig. 52.1D–F) on the postcontrast T1-weighted study.

DIAGNOSIS

Subarachnoid cysticercosis.

DISCUSSION

Neurocysticercosis is the most common parasitic central nervous system (CNS) infection in the world. The infection is caused by the *Taenia solium* parasite (pork tapeworm). This parasite is endemic in Asia, Central and South America, Africa, and Mexico. Its incidence is rapidly increasing in North America. The larval form of the tapeworm is the agent responsible for CNS cysticercosis. Humans are the definitive host of the tapeworm *T. solium* and usually harbor the adult tapeworm in the small intestine as an asymptomatic infestation. Eggs are shed by the definitive host (humans) in the feces and are then ingested (usually via contaminated water or food) by the intermediate host (typically pigs or humans). Once in the intestine, the eggs release oncospheres, the primary larvae. The primary larvae bore through the intestinal wall and enter the bloodstream. There is then hematogenous spread to neural, muscular, and ocular tissues. When pigs are the intermediate host, neurocysticercosis is contracted by humans via the ingestion of oncospheres (primary larvae) in poorly cooked pork. Once in the brain, oncospheres transform into secondary larvae: the cysticerci. Cysticerci are ovoid paralytic cysts, which consist of a focal rounded collection of clear fluid (rarely greater than 1.5 cm) with central invaginated scolex or larval head. The CNS is involved in 60% to 90% of patients with cysticercosis. The identification of these cysticerci on neuroimaging is virtually pathognomonic of this disease. The cyst evokes little host reaction as long as it remains intact. Once implanted, these parasitic cysts can lie dormant for years. Eventually, however, the larvae die and there is an acute inflammatory reaction related to degeneration of the cyst, granulation tissue, and scar formation. It is this marked host response following larval death that results in the morbidity associated with neurocysticercosis. In the final stage, the cyst usually calcifies.

The brain parenchyma is the most commonly affected site in neurocysticercosis (more than 50%). Lesions are typically found at the corticomedullary junction. Intraventricular cysticercosis is found in 20% to 50% of cases. The fourth ventricle is the most common site. Neurocysticercosis is rarely isolated to the subarachnoid space (shown in this case) and is seen in only 10% of cases. More than one anatomic site is usually involved.

Clinically, patients typically present with seizures (50% to 70%), headache, signs of intracranial hypertension, and/or focal neurological deficit.

On imaging, there are four patterns of disease that reflect the pathology of, and host response to, neurocysticercosis. These include the vesicular, colloidal vesicular, granular nodular, and nodular calcified stage. During the first stage (vesicular stage), the secondary larva (cysticercus) consists of a thin capsule surrounding a viable larva, and its fluid-containing bladder. On neuroimaging, the cysticercus appears as a round CSF signal cyst with an intermediate signal eccentric nodule that represents the scolex (or larval head) (see Case 20). The scolex is often best seen on fluid-attenuated inversion-recovery or proton density acquisition. Perifocal edema and enhancement are extremely rare. The colloidal vesicular stage represents the death and degeneration of the larva, prompting an acute inflammatory response. The host forms a thickened fibrous capsule with resultant parenchymal edema with ring (two thirds of cases) or nodular-type enhancement. Cyst fluid is hyperintense/hyperdense on MRI and CT, respectively. During the granular nodular stage, the cyst retracts and forms a nodule, which will even-

tually calcify. Occasionally, the scolex is calcified at this stage. The cysts are isodense on CT with or without central calcification. The lesion is typically isointense on T1-weighted images and isointense to hypointense on T2-weighted acquisition. Nodular or micro ring enhancement is common at this stage, suggestive of granuloma. Perifocal edema persists. The final stage is the nodular calcified stage in which the lesion has shrunk and become mineralized. On CT, there are single or multiple calcified nodules. On MRI, the lesions are hypointense on all pulse sequences. Lesions are most conspicuous on gradient echo acquisition. Typically, there is little or no edema or enhancement in this stage. Enhancement of calcified nodules in the nodular calcified stage has, however, been reported. The presence of parenchymal brain calcifications on CT studies has been identified as the only independent factor directly related to seizure recurrence after cysticidal therapy. The presence of persistent enhancement of calcified lesions may be an additional risk factor for posttreatment seizures.

Intraventricular cysticercosis accounts for 20% to 50% of neurocysticercosis. As in the parenchymal form, the status of the larva determines the imaging findings. A dying intraventricular larva results in ventriculitis. Most often, intraventricular cysts are unattached and freely mobile. As a result, they can cause intermittent or positional obstruction of the ventricular system with potential for sudden death, highlighting the importance of their detection. In contradistinction to parenchymal cysts, intraventricular cysts very rarely calcify. On MRI, the cyst wall, scolex, and subependymal reaction are readily seen.

In cisternal neurocysticercosis, the subarachnoid space and meninges are involved. It is rare as an isolated finding and is frequently associated with parenchymal disease. Hydrocephalus is often present, either obstructive or related to basal arachnoiditis. A racemose form of subarachnoid cysticercosis features a multiloculated cyst measuring several centimeters in size. They usually occur in the basal cistern and cerebellopontine angle and can simulate low-density tumors. Subarachnoid cysticerci are unique in that they lack a scolex.

Involvement of the spinal canal, seen in another case as a large cystic intradural mass within the lumbar spine on axial T1-weighted (Fig. 52.1G) and sagittal T2-weighted image (Fig. 52.1H), is thought to be the result of direct CSF dissemination of the larvae via the subarachnoid space from the cerebrum. They present as intradural extramedullary cysts or as arachnoiditis. Intramedullary cysticercosis is extremely rare but has been reported.

SUGGESTED READING

Noujaim SE, Rossi MD, Rao SK, et al. CT and MR imaging of neurocysticercosis. *AJR* 1999;173:1,485–1,490.

Osborn AG. Infections of the brain and its linings. In: *Diagnostic neuroradiology,* 1st ed. St. Louis: Mosby, 1994:708–709.

Rhee RS, Kumasaki DY, Sarwar M, et al. MR imaging of intraventricular cysticercosis. *JCAT* 1987;11(4):598–601.

Sheth TN, Pilon L, Keystone J, et al. Persistent MR contrast enhancement of calcified neurocysticercosis lesions. *AJNR* 1998;19:79–82.

Suss RA, Maravilla KR, Thompson J. MR imaging of intracranial cysticercosis: comparison with CT and anatomopathologic features. *AJNR* 1986;7:235–242.

Zee C, Segall HD, Boswell W, et al. MR imaging of neurocysticercosis. *JCAT* 1988;12(6):927–934.

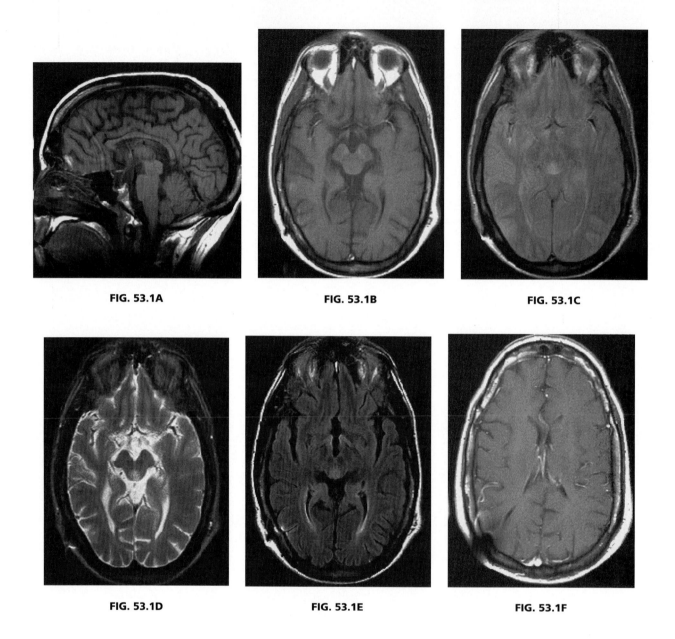

FIG. 53.1A   **FIG. 53.1B**   **FIG. 53.1C**

FIG. 53.1D   **FIG. 53.1E**   **FIG. 53.1F**

CLINICAL HISTORY

A 19-year-old man with chronic headaches and recent onset of mild gait disturbance.

FINDINGS

A mass is evident within the tectum measuring $2 \times 1 \times 1$ cm^3. It is hypointense on the T1-weighted image and does not enhance (Fig. 53.1A and B). T2 hyperintensity is seen within the lesion on the dual echo and fluid-attenuated inversion-recovery images (Fig. 53.1C–E). A ventricular shunt is present (Fig. 53.1F) for treatment of the associated obstructive hydrocephalus. *Submitted by Peter Brotchie, M.B.B.S., Ph.D., Sattam Lingawi, M.B., Ch.B., F.R.C.P.C., and William G. Bradley, M.D., Ph.D., F.A.C.R., Senior Editor, Long Beach Memorial Medical Center, Long Beach, California.*

DIAGNOSIS

Tectal glioma.

DISCUSSION

Brainstem gliomas are usually tumors of childhood, although they can occur at any age. They have a bimodal age distribution with the second peak in the fourth decade. They constitute 10% of all pediatric intracranial tumors. Tumors involving the tectal region of the midbrain have an indolent clinical course. The close proximity to the aqueduct of Sylvius is responsible for the occurrence of hydrocephalus. Tectal tumors are usually well-circumscribed low-grade astrocytomas that may produce a dorsally exophytic mass. Prior to MRI, they may have been underdiagnosed. Controversy exists regarding the optimum management of these lesions; however, radiotherapy represents the main form of treatment.

The MRI appearance may help in determining the likelihood of disease progression and help to direct therapy. Enhancement generally indicates a higher grade of tumor. Because pathological confirmation is often difficult to obtain in these cases, MRI becomes crucially important in making the diagnosis and ruling out other entities such as multiple sclerosis and vascular malformations.

SUGGESTED READING

Landolfi JC, Thaler HT, DeAngelis LM. Adult brainstem gliomas. *Neurology* 1998;51:1,136–1,139.

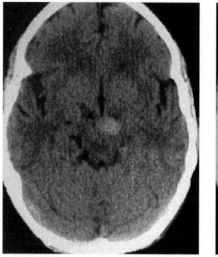

FIG. 54.1A   **FIG. 54.1B**

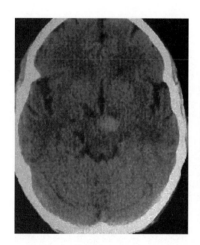

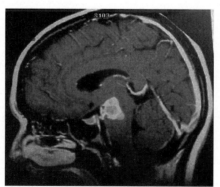

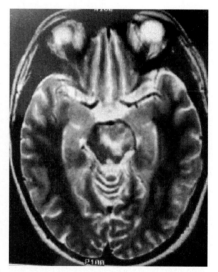

FIG. 54.1C   **FIG. 54.1D**   **FIG. 54.1E**

CLINICAL HISTORY

A 26-year-old woman presented with a sudden onset of diplopia, ataxia, and bilateral ptosis. The left eye showed a sluggishly reactive 5-mm pupil, as well as decreased abduction and upward gaze. The right eye had a briskly reactive 4-mm pupil and a normal range of ocular motion. Mild bilateral upper extremity hyperreflexia was also present.

FINDINGS

Nonenhanced CT scan of the head reveals a $2 \times 2 \times 2$ cm^3 solid hyperdense intraaxial mass expanding the left cerebral peduncle and effacing the interpeduncular cistern (Fig. 54.1A). No calcification is demonstrated. Contrast-enhanced CT scan demonstrated mildly heterogeneous pattern of enhancement with no definite areas of necrosis (Fig. 54.1B). No meningeal enhancement is demonstrated. On T1-weighted imaging, the mass has low signal (Fig. 54.1C)

with a heterogeneous pattern of enhancement and no evidence of meningeal involvement (Fig. 54.1D). The T2-weighted spin echo sequence reveals heterogeneous high signal of the lesion with no significant vasogenic edema (Fig. 54.1E). *Submitted by Sattam Lingawi, M.B., Ch.B., F.R.C.P.C., Peter Brotchie, M.B.B.S., Ph.D., and William G. Bradley, M.D., Ph.D., F.A.C.R., Senior Editor, Long Beach Memorial Medical Center, Long Beach, California.*

DIAGNOSIS

Primary rhabdomyosarcoma of the brainstem.

DISCUSSION

In adults, primary rhabdomyosarcoma of the head and neck region is most commonly seen in the paranasal sinus, particularly ethmoid and maxillary. The behavior of these tumors appears to be different in adults than in children. Although intracranial extension of head and neck rhabdomyosarcoma is not infrequent, primary intracranial sarcomas are very rare.

Primary intracranial rhabdomyosarcoma is a tumor of young patients, with no sex predominance. The tumor primarily arises in the posterior fossa. This tumor can arise primarily within the meninges without involvement of the brain parenchyma, in the parenchyma without meningeal involvement, or with both intraaxial and extraaxial involvement. In the primarily intraaxial rhabdomyosarcoma, the meningeal involvement could be secondary to contiguous invasion of the overlying meninges or to cerebrospinal fluid metastasis to the spinal leptomeninges. The absence of the

vasogenic edema and the central necrosis indicates the slow growth of the tumor and explains the large size of most of the reported cases.

Histologically, primary intracranial rhabdomyosarcomas are similar to rhabdomyosarcomas elsewhere in the body; both have rhabdomyoblasts with prominent eosinophilic cytoplasm. Since presence of rhabdomyoblasts is not uncommon in primitive neuroectodermal tumors and other undifferentiated intracranial tumors, light microscopy alone can be misleading. Immunohistochemical staining for rhabdomyoblast-specific proteins such as dismen and muscle actin, in combination with the electron microscopic demonstration of Z lines, is the most reliable method of diagnosis.

Early and accurate diagnosis is necessary for optimal prognosis. Unfortunately, most reported cases, however, have a dismal prognosis with a survival rate of less than 1 year.

SUGGESTED READING

Celli P, Cervoni L, Maraglino C. Primary rhabdomyosarcoma of the brain: observations on a case either clinical and radiological evidence of cure. *J Neuro-Oncol* 1998;36:259–267.

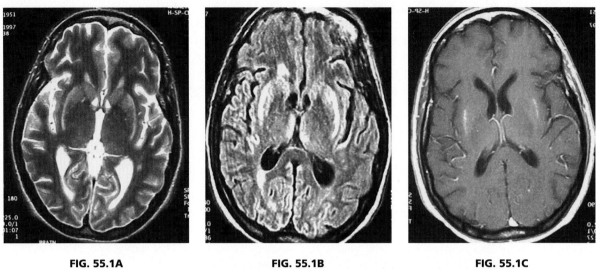

FIG. 55.1A   **FIG. 55.1B**   **FIG. 55.1C**

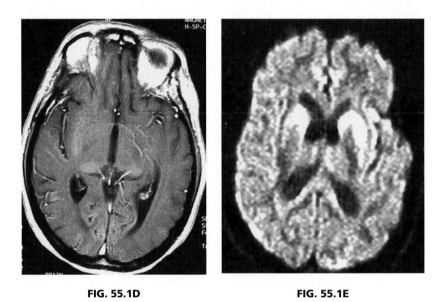

FIG. 55.1D   **FIG. 55.1E**

CLINICAL HISTORY

A 46-year-old woman who suffered a cardiac arrest following surgery.

FINDINGS

Axial T2-weighted and fluid-attenuated inversion-recovery images (Fig. 55.1A and B) demonstrate diffuse abnormal high signal within the basal ganglia bilaterally. There is subtle hyperintensity involving the thalami. Following intravenous contrast (Fig. 55.1C and D), there is patchy enhancement of the basal ganglia and thalami. Diffusion-weighted imaging (Fig. 55.1E) also shows hyperintensity involving the basal ganglia and thalami consistent with an acute ischemic event.

DIAGNOSIS

Hypoxic ischemic encephalopathy (HIE).

DISCUSSION

The high metabolic rate of neurons within the basal ganglia confers upon these structures selective vulnerability to global ischemic insults such as those suffered with cardiac arrest, asphyxiation, mishaps during anesthesia, and other sources of hypoxia. The deep layer of the cortical gray matter ribbon can also be affected, layer 5 of the cortex containing the most highly metabolic neurons.

Signal intensity elevation is caused by the increased water content associated with such insults. Subtle enhancement following intravenous contrast injection is due to early breakdown of the blood–brain barrier, the relatively tight extracellular space in these regions precluding development of large zones of vasogenic edema in the early stages. Differential diagnosis includes vascular ischemia, and metabolic conditions (especially mitochondrial cytopathies). Rarely, extrapontine myelinolysis can produce lesions in the basal ganglia simulating HIE.

SUGGESTED READING

Ginsberg MD, Hedley-Whyte E, Richardson EP Jr. Hypoxic-ischemic leukoencephalopathy in man. *Arch Neurol* 1976;33:5–14.

Mathews VP, Barker PB, Bryan RN. Magnetic resonance evaluation of stroke. *MRQ* 1992;8(4):245–263.

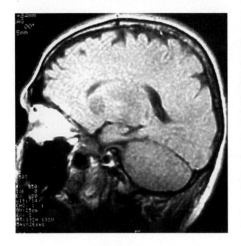

FIG. 56.1A

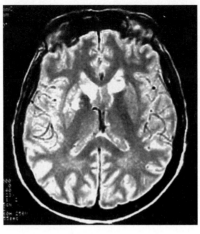

FIG. 56.1B

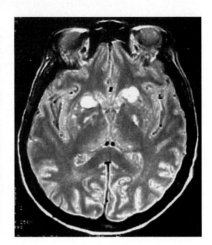

FIG. 56.1C

CLINICAL HISTORY

A 50-year-old man with recent change in mental status.

FINDINGS

Sagittal T1-weighted acquisition (Fig. 56.1A) demonstrates a large hypointense lesion within the basal ganglia. Axial proton density images (Fig. 56.1B and C) show multifocal, lobulated hyperintense lesions within the basal ganglia bilaterally. No cortical lesions are identified.

DIAGNOSIS

Cryptococcosis in a nonimmunocompromised patient.

DISCUSSION

Cryptococcal disease is the most common fungal disease to involve the central nervous system (CNS). A significant percentage of cryptococcal CNS infections today are seen in the acquired immunodeficiency syndrome (AIDS) population. Other predisposing disorders include diabetes mellitus, malignant neoplasm, renal disease, collagen vascular disease, alcoholism, and other immunocompromised patients such as patients on corticosteroids and cytotoxic chemotherapy. Cryptococcus ranks third after human immunodeficiency virus and *Toxoplasma gondii* on the list of infectious agents causing CNS disease in patients with AIDS. Cryptococcosis is a subacute granulomatous meningitis caused by *Cryptococcus neoformans*. Headache is the most common and sometimes the only manifestation. Other clinical findings include fever, seizures, and rarely focal neurological deficits.

In contrast to other fungal disease, cryptococcal disease incites little to no inflammatory response. The most common radiologic finding in patients with cryptococcal meningitis is a normal CT and MRI scan. A frequently described characteristic, but not a pathognomonic finding, is multiple symmetric well-defined hyperintense lesions at the base of the brain, known as "gelatinous pseudocysts." The hyperintense masses are best seen on intermediate and T2-weighted images (following cerebrospinal fluid signal). Pseudocysts are subtle hypodense or hypointense to isointense lesions on CT and T1-weighted MRI, respectively. There is little to no host response as demonstrated by lack of contrast enhancement or perifocal edema.

Pathologically, the lesions correspond to nests of cryptococcal organisms, which extend from the basal cisterns through the perivascular spaces (Virchow-Robin spaces), along the deep perforating arteries of the brain. There is resultant dilation of the perivascular subarachnoid space. Additionally, these organisms produce a mucoidlike material, which contributes to the formation of these fluid signal masses. The lesions are ultimately found in the basal ganglia, internal capsule, thalamus, and brainstem. Gelatinous pseudocysts are classically described in AIDS patients with cryptococcal meningitis; however, they have been described in non-AIDS patients with cryptococcal meningitis. Widening of the basal cisterns, ventricles, and sulci has been reported in CNS cryptococcosis. This may in part be due to a communicating or obstructive hydrocephalus related to the meningitis; however, it is more likely related to atrophy, particularly in the AIDS population. Enhancing mass lesions, known as "cryptococcomas," have also been described. They can occur at the base of the brain by direct invasion of fungi into the brain parenchyma from the perivascular spaces or in the cortex due to parenchymal invasion from overlying meningeal disease. A diffuse miliary pattern of enhancement (involving parenchyma and leptomeninges) has been reported.

The primary differential diagnosis for multifocal basal ganglia lesions is multiple lacunar infarcts. Toxoplasmosis and lymphoma have a predilection for the deep gray matter, but they usually enhance. Other opportunistic infectious agents to consider are cysticercosis or echinococcosis. These lesions may or may not enhance but often calcify.

SUGGESTED READING

Mathews VP, Alo PL, Glass JD, et al. AIDS-related CNS cryptococcosis: radiologic-pathologic correlation. *AJNR* 1992;13:1,477–1,486.

Sze G, Brant-Zawadzki MN, Norman D, et al. The neuroradiology of AIDS. *Semin Roentgenol* 1987;22(1):42–53.

Tien RD, Chu PK, Hesselink JR, et al. Intracranial cryptococcosis in immunocompromised patients: CT and MR findings in 29 cases. *AJNR* 1991;12:283–289.

Wehn SM, Heinz ER, Burger PC, et al. Dilated Virchow-Robin spaces in cryptococcal meningitis associated with AIDS: CT and MR findings. *JCAT* 1989;13(5):756–762.

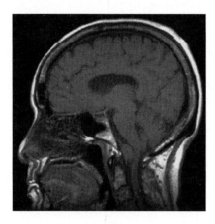

FIG. 57.1A

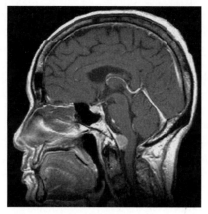

FIG. 57.1B

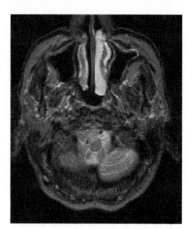

FIG. 57.1C

CLINICAL HISTORY

A 42-year-old woman with a history of slowly progressive bilateral leg weakness over 1 year. On neurological examination, the patient had mild bilateral lower extremity weakness, spasticity, and positive Babinski sign.

FINDINGS

There is a well-defined extraaxial solid mass in the anterior subarachnoid space at the level of the foramen magnum. Widening of the surrounding cerebrospinal fluid spaces confirms the intradural, extramedullary location of the mass. The mass is isointense to gray matter on T1-weighted (Fig. 57.1A) and T2-weighted (Fig. 57.1C) images. Mass effect with compression and deformity of the adjacent brainstem (upper medulla) is well demonstrated. The lesion demonstrates a homogenous pattern of enhancement following gadolinium administration (Fig. 57.1B) with a dural tail on its superior border. There is no evidence of cystic change or necrosis and no intraaxial signal abnormality is present. *Submitted by Peter Brotchie, M.B.B.S., Ph.D., Sattam Lingawi, M.B., Ch.B., F.R.C.P.C., and William G. Bradley, M.D., Ph.D., F.A.C.R., Senior Editor, Long Beach Memorial Medical Center, Long Beach, California.*

DIAGNOSIS

Foramen magnum meningioma.

DISCUSSION

Meningiomas constitute most (70%) tumors arising at the foramen magnum. They comprise 6% to 7% of all posterior fossa meningiomas and have an overall incidence rate of 1.8%. Similar to meningiomas in other intracranial sites, meningiomas in the foramen magnum also show female predominance. This location leads to often unrecognized insidiously progressive symptomatology, which may even have a remitting pattern suggestive of multiple sclerosis. The deep location of these tumors surrounded by some of the most critical structures of the nervous system, together with their potential for cure, makes them a formidable surgical challenge.

Although there is no classical syndrome of foramen magnum meningiomas, a group of certain findings with variable clinical courses can be discerned. Patients often complain of an occipital or upper cervical deeply seated pain that is accentuated by neck movement and straining. This is occasionally misdiagnosed as cervical spondylosis. As the tumor enlarges, compression of the upper medulla and the lower cranial nerves develops gradually and progressively. This results in the development of variable sensory and motor deficits. These include dysesthesia, hypesthesia, and asymmetrical quadriparesis.

MRI has become the modality of choice for imaging foramen magnum abnormalities. Accurate evaluation of the tumor location, extension, attachment, and the involvement of adjacent structures is of utmost importance in the surgical planning of the best approach. Vertebral angiography with test occlusion is occasionally performed preoperatively to assess the feasibility of unilateral vertebral artery sacrifice if necessary.

SUGGESTED READING

David CA, Spetzler RF. Foramen magnum meningiomas. *Clin Neurosurg* 1997;44:467–489.
George B, Lot G, Boissonnet H. Meningioma of the foramen magnum: a series of 40 cases. *Surg Neurol* 1997;47:371–379.

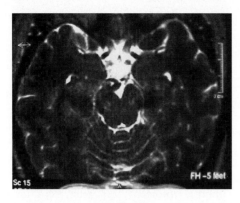

FIG. 58.1A

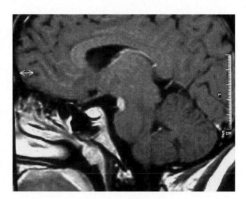

FIG. 58.1B

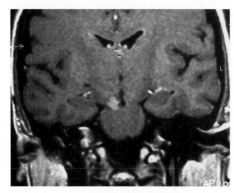

FIG. 58.1C

FIG. 58.1D

CLINICAL HISTORY

A 53-year-old man presented with persistent headache and diplopia.

FINDINGS

A 5-mm solid mass is seen arising from the cisternal segment of the oculomotor nerve. The mass is hypointense on T2-weighted images (Fig. 58.1A) and enhances strongly and homogeneously after gadolinium administration (Fig. 58.1B and C). The sagittal image demonstrates the attachment of the lesion to the oculomotor nerve (Fig. 58.1D). *Submitted by Sattam Lingawi, M.B., Ch.B., F.R.C.P.C., Peter Brotchie, M.B.B.S., Ph.D., F.R.C.P.C., William G. Bradley, M.D., Ph.D., F.A.C.R., Senior Editor, Long Beach Memorial Medical Center, Long Beach, California.*

DIAGNOSIS

Schwannoma of the oculomotor nerve.

DISCUSSION

Schwannomas account for 8% to 10% of primary intracranial tumors. Most schwannomas arise from sensory nerves, with the superior division of the vestibular nerve being the most common site. However, schwannomas of the oculomotor nerve are very rare in patients without neurofibromatosis. Only 17 cases of isolated oculomotor nerve schwannomas have been reported in the literature.

The nuclei for the oculomotor nerves (cranial nerve III) are located in the periaqueductal gray matter of the midbrain. The nerve passes ventrally through the red nucleus and exits the brainstem from the medial aspect of the cerebral peduncle into the interpeduncular cistern. It courses anteriorly and passes through the lateral wall of the cavernous sinus. Eventually, the nerve enters the orbit through the superior orbital fissure and supplies all extraocular muscles, except the lateral rectus and the superior oblique.

MRI is considered the diagnostic method of choice for visualization and evaluation of cranial nerve abnormalities. Typically cranial nerve schwannomas appear hypointense to brainstem on T1-weighted and hyperintense on T2-weighted images. Calcifications and cystic changes are commonly seen in schwannomas, which result in a heterogeneous appearance. Gadolinium-enhanced dynamic MRI reveals a pattern of gradual increase in intensity of schwannomas. In comparison, meningiomas show a strong early enhancement with prolonged slow contrast release. They also have a greater tendency for calcification and less of a tendency for cystic change.

The differential diagnosis includes meningiomas, lymphoma, leptomeningeal metastasis, and inflammatory conditions such as sarcoidosis.

SUGGESTED READING

Katsuyuki A, Sawamura Y, Murai H, et al. Schwannoma of the oculomotor nerve: a case report with consideration of the surgical treatment. *Neurosurgery* 1999;45:630–634.

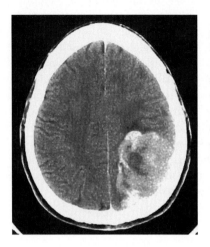

FIG. 59.1A

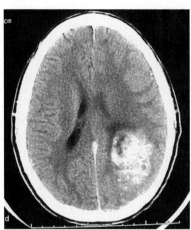

FIG. 59.1B

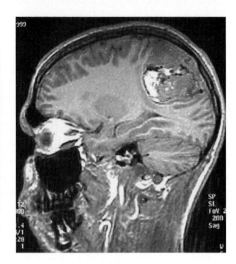

FIG. 59.1C

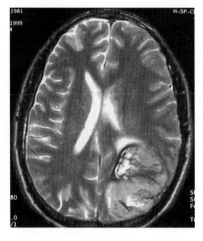

FIG. 59.1D

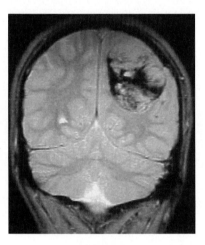

FIG. 59.1E

CLINICAL HISTORY

An 18-year-old man with first seizure, recent mild head trauma.

FINDINGS

Noncontrast axial CT image (Fig. 59.1A and B) demonstrates a large well-defined, lobulated mass within the left parietal lobe with areas of high and low density consistent with a large hemorrhagic and/or calcified mass. Sagittal T1-acquisition (Fig. 59.1C) shows a large heterogeneous intraaxial mass within the left parietal lobe with foci of high signal consistent with subacute blood. There are also foci of very low signal on all pulse sequences con-sistent with calcification or hemosiderin deposition. Axial T2-weighted acquisition (Fig. 59.1D) shows patchy regions of high signal consistent with extracellular methemoglobin. Magnetic susceptibility effects of the associated blood products are well demonstrated on the coronal gradient echo image (Fig. 59.1E). There is perilesional edema with associated mass effect effacing the left lateral ventricle and cortical sulci.

DIAGNOSIS

Primitive neuroectodermal tumor (PNET).

DISCUSSION

PNETs comprise a group of tumors thought to originate from primitive or undifferentiated neuroepithelial cells, which display the capacity to differentiate along both glial and neuronal lines. There remains controversy regarding the classification of PNETs. The prototype of these tumors is the medulloblastoma, which accounts for 85% of PNETs and arises in the posterior fossa. Other tumors designated as PNETs include cerebral neuroblastoma, pineoblastoma, spongioblastoma, ependymoblastoma, and medulloepithelioma. Supratentorial PNETs account for less than 1% of pediatric brain tumors. Eighty-five percent of these tumors occur before the age of 10 while sixty-five percent occur before 5 years of age. The most common location for supratentorial PNET is the frontal lobes, followed by the parietal, temporal, and occipital lobes. They can even be intraventricular. Approximately 50% to 70% of supratentorial PNETs contain calcium, a much higher percentage than infratentorial PNETs (or medulloblastoma).

Histologically, PNETs are dense, hypercellular tumors primarily composed of small cells with scant cytoplasm. It is the dense cellularity and high nuclear-cytoplasmic ratio that is thought to account for their unique intermediate to low signal on T2-weighted acquisition. On CT, they are typically heterogeneous, high-density, well-circumscribed masses. On MRI, PNETs are described as large heterogeneous masses with very little edema relative to their size. Foci of calcification, hemorrhage, and cystic change are frequently present. The solid portion of the mass typically enhances. Hydrocephalus may be present. Differential diagnosis for large heterogeneous enhancing supratentorial mass includes PNET, ependymoma, oligodendroglioma, and glioblastoma multiforme glomerular basement membrane (GBM).

SUGGESTED READING

Rorke LB, Trojanowski JQ, Lee VM, et al. Primitive neuroectodermal tumors of the central nervous system. *Brain Pathol* 1997;7:765–784.

Davis PC, Wichman RD, Takei Y, et al. Primary cerebral neuroblastoma: CT and MR findings in 12 cases. *AJNR* 1990;11:115–120.

Luh GY, Bird CR. Imaging of brain tumors in the pediatric population. *Neuroimaging Clin North Am* 1999;9(4):691–716.

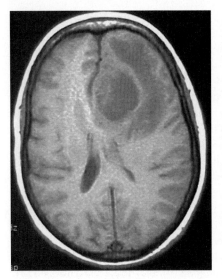

FIG. 60.1A

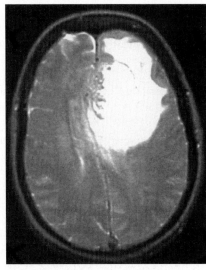

FIG. 60.1B

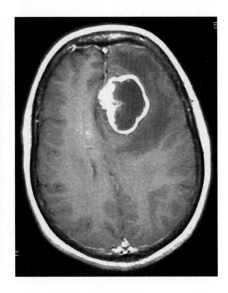

FIG. 60.1C

CLINICAL HISTORY

A 53-year-old woman with right-sided weakness and altered behavior.

FINDINGS

Axial T1-weighted and T2-weighted images (Fig. 60.1A and B) show a large mass lesion within the parasagittal left frontal lobe. The lesion has intermediate signal in its rim, with central hypointensity on the T1-weighted acquisition that becomes hyperintense on the T2-weighted image. There is significant perifocal edema. The lesion abuts the left lateral ventricle and causes effacement of the frontal horn and displacement of the midline structures toward the right. T2-weighted images demonstrate no abnormal signal within the corpus callosum or right cerebral hemisphere. Following intravenous contrast (Fig. 60.1C), the T1-weighted image shows peripheral enhancement with a central nonenhancing region consistent with necrosis.

DIAGNOSIS

Malignant ependymoma.

DISCUSSION

Ependymomas are glial neoplasms derived from ependymal cells that line the ventricles and central canal of the spinal cord. Ependymal cell rests within the white matter account for extraventricular ependymomas, as seen in this case. Approximately 40% of ependymomas are supratentorial. Most supratentorial ependymomas are extraventricular as opposed to infratentorial tumors, which are typically within the fourth ventricle (90%). The average age at presentation is 16 to 24 years (infratentorial ependymomas have two age peaks at 5 years and 35 years). Overall, ependymomas are malignant in approximately 70% of cases. Metastasis along the cerebrospinal fluid pathways occurs in 10% to 20% of infratentorial tumors. Metastasis is rare in supratentorial ependymoma. When metastases occur in supratentorial ependymoma, they are supratentorial. In infratentorial tumor, metastasis is usually intraspinal.

Supratentorial ependymomas usually appear as mixed solid and cystic masses. Parenchymal tumors are usually in close proximity to a ventricular surface. The solid portions of the mass are typically isointense to hypointense to brain on T1-weighted images and hyperintense on T2-weighted images. Occasionally, intrinsic hemorrhage leads to hyperintensity on T1-weighted images. Heterogeneous signal reflects hemosiderin, methemoglobin, necrosis, and calcification or cyst formation. Enhancement pattern may be solid or ring enhancing. On CT, ependymomas are mixed density masses, often with foci of calcification (50%). Supratentorial ependymomas are often indistinguishable from other gliomas. Biopsy is necessary for definitive diagnosis. The mainstay of treatment for intracranial ependymoma is surgical excision. Lesion location, histologic degree of malignancy, and adjuvant chemotherapy have no impact on survival. Studies show it is the extent of surgical excision, as determined by the operative report and postoperative imaging studies, that is the most important determinant of long-term outcome. The 5-year survival rate in patients with total or near-total excision is approximately 64%.

SUGGESTED READING

Coulon RA, Till K. Intracranial ependymomas in children: a review of 43 cases. *Childs Brain* 1977;3:154–168.

Furie DM, Provencale JM. Supratentorial ependymoma and subependymoma: CT and MR appearance. *JCAT* 1995;19(4):518–526.

Osborn AG. Astrocytomas and other glial neoplasms. In: *Diagnostic Neuroradiology,* 1st ed. St. Louis: Mosby, 1994:566–570.

Spoto GP, Press GA, Hesselink JR, et al. Intracranial ependymoma and subependymoma: MR manifestations. *AJR* 1990;154(4):837–845.

Sutton W, Goldwein J, Perilongo G, et al. Prognostic factors in childhood ependymoma. *Pediatr Neurosurg* 1990–91;16(2):57–65.

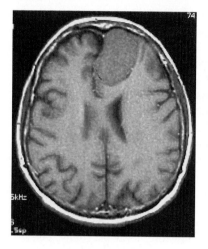

FIG. 61.1A

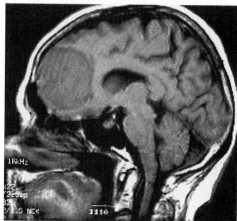

FIG. 61.1B

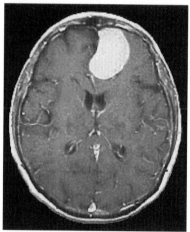
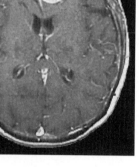

FIG. 61.1C

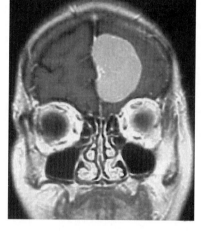

FIG . 61.1D

CLINICAL HISTORY

A 53-year-old woman with 1-year history of morning headaches, personality changes, and bilateral anosmia.

FINDINGS

A large (5 × 5 × 4 cm³), well-defined, solid, extraaxial mass is present in the left frontopolar region, abutting the anterior falx. The mass is isointense to brain parenchyma on the T1-weighted images (Fig. 61.1A and B) and enhances homogeneously (Fig. 61.1C and D). No cystic change or necrosis is detected. Despite the significant mass effect on the adjacent frontal lobe parenchyma and the frontal horns of the lateral ventricles (with midline shift), no parenchymal edema is detected. *Submitted by Sattam Lingawi, M.B., Ch.B., F.R.C.P.C., Peter Brotchie, M.B.B.S., Ph.D., F.R.C.P.C., and William G. Bradley, M.D., Ph.D., F.A.C.R., Senior Editor, Long Beach Memorial Medical Center, Long Beach, California.*

DIAGNOSIS

Frontal meningioma.

DISCUSSION

Meningiomas are the most common intracranial extraaxial tumor in adults. There is a particular predilection for middle-aged women. Multiple meningiomas are uncommon and tend to occur in type II neurofibromatosis. Although meningiomas can occur anywhere in the brain, 50% are parasagittal in location. Other common locations include the sphenoid wing (20%), the olfactory groove (10%), the parasellar region (10%), the cerebellopontine angle, the posterior fossa, and the foramen magnum. On MRI, they are usually isointense to brain parenchyma on T1-weighted and T2-weighted images. The relative low intensity of meningiomas on T2-weighted images compared to that of gliomas is believed to be due to reduced water content and psammomatous calcification. Gadolinium classically results in early, strong, and homogenous enhancement of the tumor and may reveal a dural tail, which is highly suggestive of, but not pathognomonic for, this entity. Due to the slow growth rate of these tumors, they often achieve large size with minimal or no symptoms. Vasogenic edema in the adjacent parenchyma may be present and is thought to be secondary to compression or invasion of adjacent cortical veins and dural venous sinuses. Hyperostosis of the adjacent bony structures is present in 5% of cases and is best evaluated with CT. Patient symptomatology depends primarily on the tumor location. Thus, these tumors are often discovered incidentally or may cause vague symptoms such as headache.

SUGGESTED READING

Buetow MAP, Buetow PC, Smirniotopoulos DG. Typical, atypical and misleading features in meningioma. *Radiographics* 1991;11:1,087.

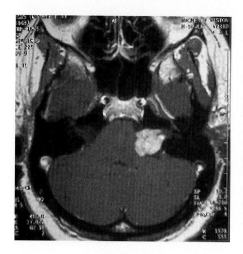

FIG. 62.1A

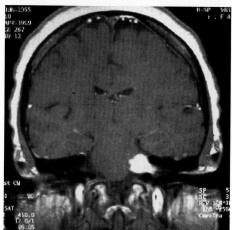

FIG. 62.1B

CLINICAL HISTORY

A 61-year-old man with left-sided sensorineural hearing loss.

FINDINGS

A large well-defined, solid extraaxial mass is present in the left cerebellopontine angle on the T1-weighted images, enhancing homogeneously (Fig. 62.1A and B). The mass displaces the pons to the right with enlargement of the cerebellopontine angle cistern on the left and extends into the left internal auditory canal. *Submitted by Peter Brotchie, M.B.B.S., Ph.D., Sattam Lingawi, M.B., Ch.B., F.R.C.P.C., and William G. Bradley, M.D., Ph.D., F.A.C.R., Senior Editor, Long Beach Memorial Medical Center, Long Beach, California.*

DIAGNOSIS

Vestibular schwannoma.

DISCUSSION

Acoustic neuroma (better called "vestibular schwannoma") is the most common mass in the cerebellopontine angle causing unilateral sensorineural hearing loss. It is a benign tumor of Schwann cells and usually arises from the superior division of the vestibular nerve. The tumor can be completely intracanalicular (i.e., inside the internal auditory canal), completely extracanalicular (in the cerebellopontine angle), or it can have a component of both, which results in an "ice-cream cone" appearance.

The current imaging test of choice for diagnosing vestibular schwannoma is MRI. Contrast-enhanced T1-weighted images have high sensitivity and specificity for the diagnosis of this entity but require the intravenous administration of contrast. Several studies have documented that there are no statistically significant differences in the sensitivity and specificity of high-resolution (512 × 512) T2-weighted images and contrast-enhanced T1-weighted images for the detection of acoustic schwannoma. Such techniques enable one to directly visualize the four nerves within the internal auditory canal as separate structures and subsequently minimize the possibility of false-negative or false-positive results.

The primary pathology in the differential diagnosis is the cerebellopontine angle meningioma. However, the lack of intracanalicular extension or cystic changes and the presence of a dural tail make this possibility less likely. The extent of these lesions should be carefully assessed and described because it has a direct influence on the surgical approach.

SUGGESTED READING

Fukui MB, Wiessman JL, Curtin HD, et al. T2-weighted MR characteristics of internal auditory canal masses. *AJNR* 1996; 17:1,211–1,218.

Stuckey SA, Harris AJ, Mannolini S. Detection of acoustic schwannoma: use of constructive interference in the steady state three dimensional MR. *AJNR* 1996;17:1,219–1,225.

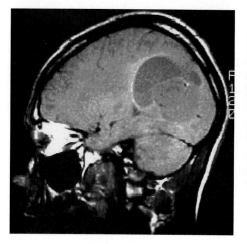

FIG. 63.1A

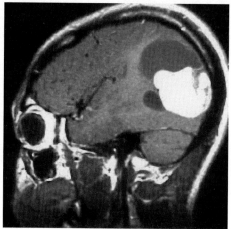

FIG. 63.1B

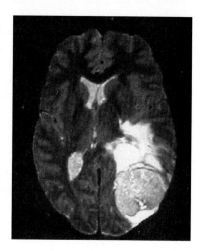

FIG. 63.1C

CLINICAL HISTORY

A 21-year-old woman with chronic, generalized seizures.

FINDINGS

A large complex mass is evident in the left parietal region with both cystic and solid components. The cystic components are somewhat brighter than cerebrospinal fluid on both T1-weighted and T2-weighted images (Fig. 63.1A and C) reflecting higher protein content. The signal characteristics of the solid nodule match those of gray matter. A moderate amount of vasogenic edema and mass effect is noted. Gadolinium administration results in strong enhancement of the nodule (Fig. 63.1B). *Submitted by Peter Brotchie, M.B.B.S., Ph.D., Sattam Lingawi, M.B., Ch.B., F.R.C.P.C., and William G. Bradley, M.D., Ph.D., F.A.C.R., Senior Editor, Long Beach Memorial Medical Center, Long Beach, California.*

DIAGNOSIS

Pleomorphic xanthoastrocytoma.

DISCUSSION

Pleomorphic xanthoastrocytoma is an uncommon but distinctive variant of astrocytoma, which was first described by Kerpes in 1979. The tumor occurs predominantly during the second and third decades of life and is most often located superficially in the cerebral hemispheres, typically the temporal or temporoparietal regions. An associated cyst is frequently present. Patients with pleomorphic xanthoastrocytoma treated surgically have a relatively good prognosis, despite the marked cellular pleomorphism that suggests a malignant glioma. In light of the frequently indolent behavior, recognition of this entity is critical to avoid overly aggressive treatment.

These tumors typically become symptomatic in childhood with seizures. It is usually only somewhat later that symptoms of mass effect appear and prompt surgery. The tumor is frequently composed of a cyst with a superficially located nodule. The nodule is usually isointense with gray matter on T1-weighted and hyperintense on T2-weighted images and shows strong enhancement with gadolinium.

The differential diagnosis for these lesions includes supratentorial pilocytic astrocytoma and ganglioglioma.

SUGGESTED READING

Kros JM, Vecht CJ, Stefanko SZ. The pleomorphic xanthoastrocytoma and its differential diagnosis: a study of five cases. *Hum Pathol* 1991;22:1,128–1,135.

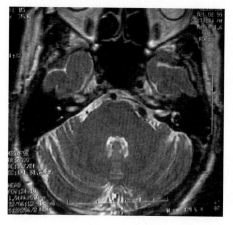

FIG. 64.1A

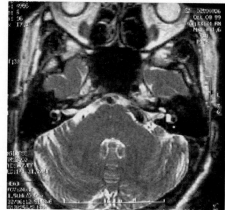

FIG. 64.1B

CLINICAL HISTORY

A 43-year-old man with left-sided hemifacial spasm.

FINDINGS

An ectatic left vertebral artery displaces the left facial nerve posteriorly (Fig. 64.1A and B). *Submitted by Sattam Lingawi, M.B., Ch.B., F.R.C.P.C., Peter Brotchie, M.B.B.S., Ph.D., and William G. Bradley, M.D., Ph.D., F.A.C.R., Senior Editor, Long Beach Memorial Medical Center, Long Beach, California.*

DIAGNOSIS

Hemifacial spasm.

DISCUSSION

Hemifacial spasm is characterized by unilateral involuntary contractions of muscles innervated by the facial nerve. It usually has a fluctuating course, with spasm that may be triggered by factors such as stress, bright light, and swallowing. It is believed to be due to abutment or compression of the facial nerve by a vascular loop. It was originally thought that in order for such vascular compression to incite symptoms, it had to occur at the root exit zone. More recent reports have demonstrated that the same symptoms can occur due to compression of the facial nerve in its cisternal or intracanalicular segments as well. Such vascular compression is usually related to a loop in the main trunk or a branch of the posterior inferior cerebellar artery, anterior inferior cerebellar artery, or vertebral artery. There is usually no signal abnormality in either the nerve or the brainstem. With recent advances in MR technology, it is currently recommended to use ultrathin (less than 1 mm) heavily T2-weighted MRI images in the axial plane through the brainstem and internal auditory canals.

Microvascular decompression for hemifacial spasm has proven a very effective and safe surgical procedure in relieving symptoms, with a success rate of 90% to 95%. This is achieved by the placement of an Ivalon sponge or a Teflon implant between the vascular loop and the nerve.

SUGGESTED READING

Kureshi SA, Wilkins RH. Posterior fossa reexploration for persistent or recurrent trigeminal neuralgia or hemifacial spasm: surgical findings and therapeutic implications. *Neurosurgery* 1998;43(5):1,111–1,117.

Lingawi SS, Bradley WG. *Thin slice MR imaging evaluation of vascular impingement of the facial nerve in patients with hemifacial spasm.* Atlanta: ASNR Annual Meeting; April 3–8, 2000. Paper 135.

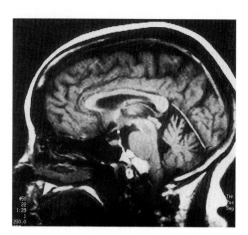

FIG. 65.1A

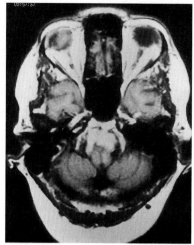

FIG. 65.1B

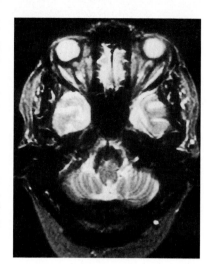

FIG. 65.1C

CLINICAL HISTORY

A 32-year-old woman presenting with severe headache 1 week earlier.

FINDINGS

High signal is noted anterior to the brainstem on the T1-weighted images (Fig. 65.1A and B), which turns dark on the T2-weighted image (Fig. 65.1C). *Submitted by William G. Bradley, M.D., Ph.D., F.A.C.R., Senior Editor, Long Beach Memorial Medical Center, Long Beach, California.*

DIAGNOSIS

Early subacute subarachnoid hematoma.

DISCUSSION

As in other compartments of the brain, early subacute hemorrhage (intracellular methemoglobin) is bright on T1-weighted images. Unlike the parenchymal compartment, however, oxidative denaturation of hemoglobin progresses more slowly in the subarachnoid space. Thus, while a 1-week-old parenchymal hematoma would almost certainly have evolved to the late subacute stage, this subarachnoid thrombosis remains in the early subacute stage with intact red cells. This reflects the higher oxygen tension in the subarachnoid space (40 mm Hg) compared to the parenchymal compartment where the oxygen tension is 20 mm Hg. Subarachnoid hematomas also differ from parenchymal hematomas in that they will never develop a hemosiderin rim (because there are no macrophages in the subarachnoid space). Larger clots will remain as subarachnoid thrombi and will eventually be resorbed.

SUGGESTED READING

Bradley WG. Hemorrhage. In: Stark DD, Bradley WG, eds. *Magnetic resonance imaging,* 3rd ed. St. Louis: Mosby, 1999.

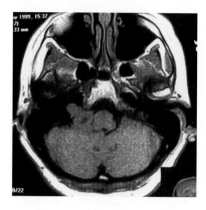

FIG. 66.1A

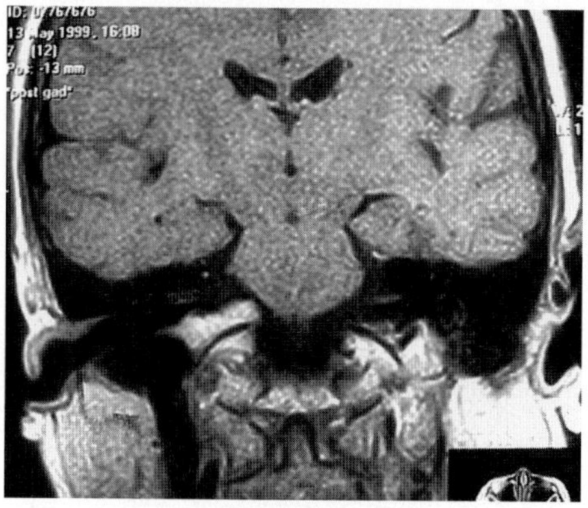

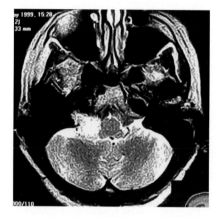

FIG. 66.1B

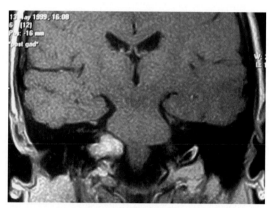

FIG. 66.1C

FIG. 66.1D

CLINICAL HISTORY

A 61-year-old woman with difficulty swallowing.

FINDINGS

Axial and coronal T1-weighted and axial T2-weighted images (Fig. 66.1A–C) show an extraaxial mass in the right cerebellar pontine angle, which is isointense to brain on T1-weighted images and heterogenous in signal on the T2-weighted acquisition. There is no involvement of the internal auditory canal. There is homogenous enhancement following contrast material (Fig. 66.1D).

DIAGNOSIS

Neuroma involving the ninth cranial nerve.

DISCUSSION

Differential diagnosis of masses in the cerebellar pontine angle includes meningioma and neuroma as the two most common causes. Most meningiomas demonstrate isointensity on T1-weighted images with isointense to slightly hyperintense signal on T2-weighted images. Neuromas, on the other hand, typically show low signal intensity on T1-weighted and homogeneous high signal intensity on T2-weighted images. Both lesions show homogeneous enhancement. Central necrosis is more typical of neuroma, whereas calcification is much more commonly shown with meningioma.

Arachnoidal adhesions creating cisternal menisci are associated with neuroma while enhancement of a dural "tail" is more commonly associated with meningioma. Involvement of the internal auditory canal, particularly flaring of its entrance, is more typical with neuroma of the acoustic nerve, whereas hyperostosis of the porous acoustics is a feature of meningioma. Occasionally, ninth nerve neuroma can simulate acoustic schwannoma, but the clinical history, the more inferior extent of the lesion, expansion of the jugular canal, and/or erosion of the jugular tubercle can help differentiate these two lesions.

The differential diagnosis includes giant aneurysm, hemangioblastoma, and metastasis. The absence of phase-related pulsation artifact, large feeding vessels, and relative lack of mass effect argue against these entities.

SUGGESTED READING

Suzuki F, Handa J, Todo G. Intracranial glosso neurinomas: report of two cases with special emphasis on CT and MR imaging findings. *Surg Neurol* 1989;31(5):390–394.

Sweasey TA, Edelstein SR, Hoff JT. Glossopharyngeal schwannoma: review of five cases and the literature. *Surg Neurol* 1991;35(2):127–130.

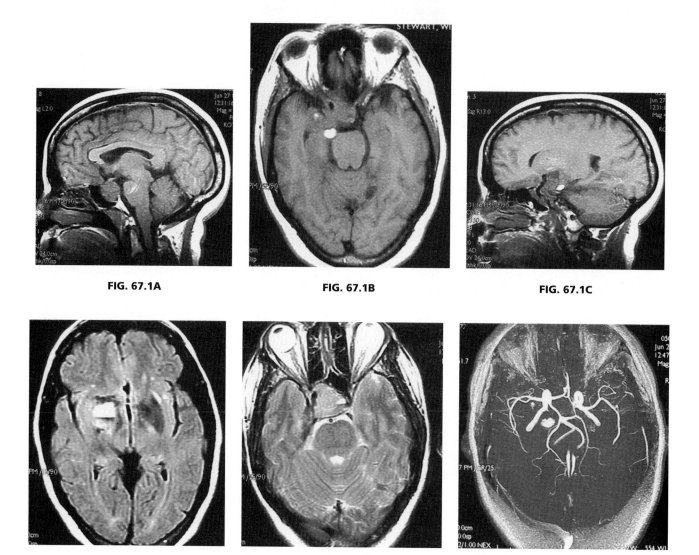

FIG. 67.1A   FIG. 67.1B   FIG. 67.1C

FIG. 67.1D   FIG. 67.1E   FIG. 67.1F

CLINICAL HISTORY

A 55-year-old woman with visual disturbance and acute onset of headache.

FINDINGS

Midline sagittal T1-weighted acquisition demonstrates a large mass within and expanding into the sella turcica (Fig. 67.1A). Axial and coronal T1-weighted (Fig. 67.1B and C) and T2-weighted images (Fig. 67.1D) show the mass to be intermediate signal on T1-weighted images and slightly hyperintense on the T2-weighted images. There is a small focus of high signal within this mass in the right parasellar region on the T1-weighted acquisition consistent with hemorrhage. A fluid level is also seen in the right parasellar region, best seen on the axial fluid-attenuated inversion-recovery image (Fig. 67.1E). Note encasement of the cavernous carotid artery due to extension of tumor into the right cavernous sinus. Collapsed view from three-dimensional time-of-flight magnetic resonance angiography of the circle of Willis (Fig. 67.1F) shows the right cavernous carotid artery is not occluded and this lesion does not arise from the circle of Willis, excluding the possibility of aneurysm. The hemorrhage is visualized in the right parasellar region due to its T1 shortening effect.

DIAGNOSIS

Hemorrhagic pituitary macroadenoma (pituitary apoplexy).

DISCUSSION

Pituitary tumors are classified by size: Those less than 10 mm are considered microadenomas and those greater than 10 mm are macroadenomas (seen in this case). Twenty-five percent of adenomas are "nonfunctioning" tumors and the remainder show clinical signs of hormone excess. In general, the hormonally active adenomas present earlier and are typically microadenomas. Macroadenomas are more often "nonfunctioning" and present with signs of mass effect on nearby structures. Rarely, an adenoma presents acutely with pituitary apoplexy (severe headache, hypotension, and sudden visual loss) because of intratumoral hemorrhage.

Pituitary adenomas are tumors of adults, as less than 10% occur in children. Pituitary macroadenoma is the most common suprasellar mass, accounting for 33% to 50% of lesions in this area.

Macroadenomas present as isodense sellar/suprasellar mass lesions on nonenhanced CT. There is moderate enhancement following contrast. One percent to eight percent of lesions calcify. On MRI, uncomplicated macroadenomas are isointense unless cystic or hemorrhagic. The characteristic configuration seen on coronal and sagittal images is a "figure-of-eight" or "snowman-shaped" mass, reflecting an intrasellar mass with suprasellar extension, the "waist," due to the relative "constriction" of the mass at the level of the diaphragma sella. The sella turcica is typically enlarged. Twenty percent to thirty percent of adenomas will demonstrate hemorrhage (seen in this case). Infarction and/or hemorrhage rarely produce the clinical syndrome of pituitary apoplexy. Most intratumoral hemorrhage is subclinical and is discovered only incidentally at imaging.

SUGGESTED READING

Elster AD. Modern imaging of the pituitary. *Radiology* 1993;187:1–14.

Johnson DE, Woodruff WW, Allen IS, et al. MR imaging of the sellar and juxtasellar regions. *Radiographics* 1991;11:727–758.

Kucharczyk W, Montanera WJ, Becker LE. The sella turcica and parasellar region. In: Atlas SW, ed. *Magnetic resonance imaging of the brain and spine,* 2nd ed. Philadelphia: Lippincott–Raven Publishers, 1996:884–894.

Kyle CA, Laster RA, Burton EM, et al. Subacute pituitary apoplexy: MR and CT appearance. *JCAT* 1990;14:40–44.

Ostrov SG, Quencer RM, Hoffman JC, et al. Hemorrhage within pituitary adenomas: how often associated with pituitary apoplexy syndrome? *AJNR* 1989;10:503–510.

Schwartzberg DG. Imaging of pituitary tumors. *Semin US Comput Tomogr Magn Reson* 1992;13:207–223.

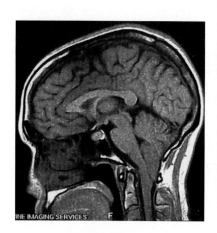

FIG. 68.1A

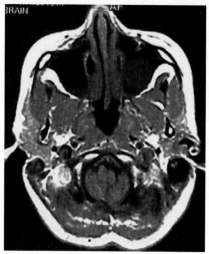

FIG. 68.1B

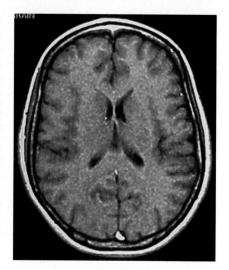

FIG. 68.1C

CLINICAL HISTORY

Headache.

FINDINGS

Sagittal T1-weighted acquisition (Fig. 68.1A) demonstrates downward displacement of the cerebellar tonsils through the foramen magnum. The tips of the cerebellar tonsils lie approximately 2 cm below the foramen magnum. They have a pointed, peglike contour inferiorly. There is a "tight" craniovertebral junction with mild compression upon the cervical medullary junction (Fig. 68.1B). Axial T1-weighted acquisition (Fig. 68.1C) shows no evidence for hydrocephalus. No parenchymal abnormality is identified.

DIAGNOSIS

Chiari I malformation.

DISCUSSION

A Chiari I malformation is a malformation of the hindbrain defined as caudal extension of the cerebellar tonsils below the foramen magnum by at least 5 mm. The herniated tonsils appear elongated, pointed, or "peglike." The degree of tonsillar ectopia is measured from a line drawn between the basion and opisthion at the skull base to the tip of the cerebellar tonsils. Children between the ages of 5 and 15 years normally have slightly greater tonsillar ectopia than adults or children less than 5 years old. In this population, tonsillar herniation is not considered pathologic unless greater than 6 mm. In all patients with Chiari I malformation, the cervical spine should be imaged to look for concurrent syringohydromyelia (seen in 20% to 25% of cases). Syrinx usually occurs between C-4 and C-6 but can involve the cervicothoracic region or the entire cord. Hydrocephalus may also be present.

Chiari I malformations are more frequent in women than men (a ratio of 3:2). Many patients are asymptomatic. Up to 30% of patients with 5 to 10 mm of tonsillar ectopia have no symptoms. Herniation greater than 12 mm is invariably symptomatic. Affected patients usually present with headache and neck pain (particularly with straining or neck flexion/extension) and cranial nerve palsies. Patients can present with a pseudotumor or Menière diseaselike syndrome. Extremity paresthesia/anesthesia symptoms can occur in patients with associated syrinx. Chiari I malformation can mimic demyelinating disease.

Most Chiari I malformations are considered congenital. Occurrence can be sporadic or familial. The primary structural abnormality is thought to be underdevelopment of the occipital bone resulting in a small overcrowded posterior fossa. The volume of the posterior fossa contents (cerebellum and brainstem) is normal; therefore, there is relative diminished cerebrospinal fluid (CSF) space, manifested radiographically as obliteration of the retrocerebellar subarachnoid space. The result is downward herniation of the cerebellar tonsils through the foramen magnum. Clinical manifestations are thought related to the subsequent CSF flow disturbance at the "tight" craniovertebral junction. Osseous anomalies are seen in about 25% of Chiari I malformation patients. These include craniovertebral dysplasias, atlantooccipital assimilation, platybasia, basilar invagination, and congenitally fused cervical vertebra (Klippel-Feil anomaly). Scoliosis has also been associated with Chiari I malformation.

Downward tonsillar herniation can be the result of increased intracranial pressure or diffuse cerebral edema due to trauma or neoplasm (see Case 86). Spontaneous intracranial hypotension or hypotension related to lumbar puncture can present in a similar fashion. In these instances, however, the tonsillar ectopia is potentially reversible (see Volume 2, Case 1).

SUGGESTED READING

Barkovich AJ. Congenital malformations of the brain and skull. In: *Pediatric neuroimaging,* 2nd ed. Philadelphia: Lippincott–Raven Publishers, 1996:238–239.

Elster AD, Chen MY. Chiari I malformation: clinical and radiologic reappraisal. *Radiology* 1992;183(2):347–353.

Milhorat TH, Chou MW, Trinidad EM, et al. Chiari I malformation redefined: clinical and radiographic findings for 364 symptomatic patients. *Neurosurgery* 1999;44(5):1,005–1,017.

Nishikawa M, Sakamoto H, Hakuba A, et al. Pathogenesis of Chiari I malformation: a morphometric study of the posterior cranial fossa. *J Neurosurg* 1997;86(1):40–47.

Osborn AG. Disorders of neural tube closure. In: *Diagnostic neuroradiology,* 1st ed. St. Louis: Mosby, 1994:16–18.

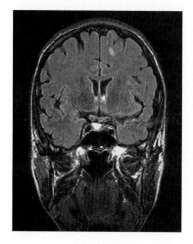

FIG. 69.1A

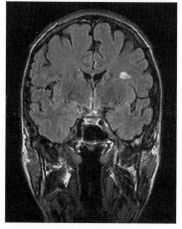

FIG. 69.1B

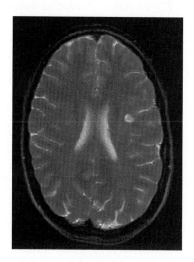

FIG. 69.1C

CLINICAL HISTORY

A 45-year-old woman with a history of systemic lupus erythematosus now presents with acute onset of confusion and decreased level of consciousness.

FINDINGS

Subcortical infarctions are present within the left frontal lobe. They have high signal on T2-weighted and fluid-attenuated inversion-recovery sequences (Fig. 69.1A–C). No surrounding edema or mass effect is detected and there is no evidence of hemorrhage. *Submitted by Peter Brotchie, M.B.B.S., Ph.D., Sattam Lingawi, M.B., Ch.B., F.R.C.P.C., and William G. Bradley, M.D., Ph.D., F.A.C.R., Senior Editor, Long Beach Memorial Medical Center, Long Beach, California.*

DIAGNOSIS

Subcortical infarctions secondary to lupus vasculitis.

DISCUSSION

Possible causes of central nervous system vasculitis include infectious, autoimmune, drug-induced, or idiopathic causes. In the autoimmune category, it is most commonly seen with systemic lupus erythematosus. Patients often present with waxing and waning focal neurological deficits. Infarctions of varying sizes and age may be present in multiple vascular territories. These generally tend to be peripheral and involve the gray-white junction. They also show a higher preponderance for hemorrhage, reflecting the weakened underlying vessels and pseudoaneurysm formation by virtue of vessel wall involvement. Cerebral angiography may demonstrate multiple foci of concentric narrowing and occlusion with downstream dilation. Atherosclerotic disease may be difficult to tell from vasculitis, however, atherosclerosis tends to produce eccentric narrowing and more often involves the carotid bifurcation and siphon. Other etiologies to consider for multiple infarctions include arterial embolism and venous occlusion. Due to the relative insensitivity of both MRI and angiography to vasculitic changes, it remains a pathological diagnosis. Because strong immunosuppressants can be of value in the treatment of this entity, brain biopsy is usually required in radiologically indeterminate cases.

The differential diagnosis of multiple enhancing lesions includes metastases, multifocal astrocytoma, lymphoma, demyelination, and infections.

SUGGESTED READING

Harris KG, Tran DD, Sickels WJ, et al. Diagnosing intracranial vasculitis: the role of MR and angiography. *AJNR* 1994;12:317.

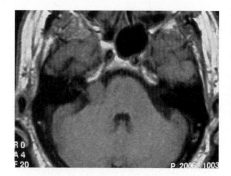

FIG. 70.1A

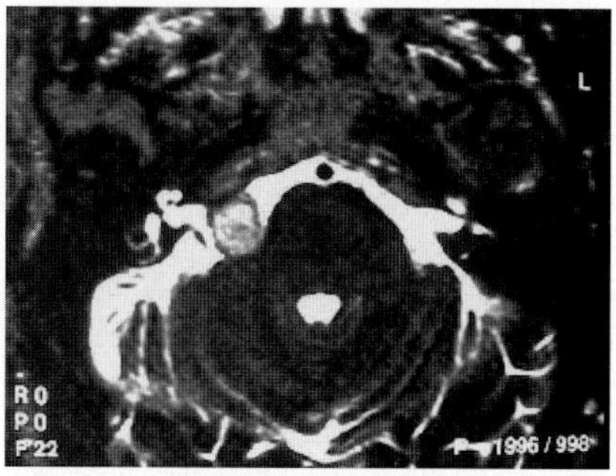

FIG. 70.1B

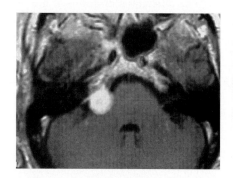

FIG. 70.1C

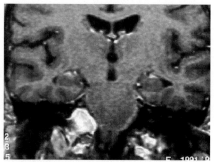

FIG. 70.1D

CLINICAL HISTORY

A 53-year-old woman complaining of headache.

FINDINGS

A 2 cm extraaxial solid mass is present in the right cerebellopontine angle. The mass is separate from the adjacent cranial nerves and the internal auditory meatus. The mass is isointense to brainstem parenchyma on T1-weighted (Fig. 70.1A) and hyperintense on T2-weighted images (Fig. 70.1B). Gadolinium-enhanced images reveal strong homogenous pattern of enhancement with a dural tail (Fig. 70.1C and D). *Submitted by Peter Brotchie, M.B.B.S., Ph.D., Sattam Lingawi, M.B., Ch.B., F.R.C.P.C., and William G. Bradley, M.D., Ph.D., F.A.C.R., Senior Editor, Long Beach Memorial Medical Center, Long Beach, California.*

DIAGNOSIS

Cerebellopontine angle meningioma.

DISCUSSION

Meningioma is the most common intracranial extraaxial tumor in adults, comprising approximately 15% of all intracranial tumors. There is a particular predilection for middle-aged women. Fifty percent of all meningiomas are parasagittal in location; however, other common locations include the sphenoid wing (20%), olfactory groove (10%), parasellar region (10%), cerebellopontine angle, posterior fossa, and foramen magnum. Gadolinium classically results in early, strong, homogenous enhancement of the tumor and may reveal a dural tail. Although a dural tail is highly suggestive of meningioma, this finding has been found in all pathological entities that come in contact with the meninges. It represents primarily a focal inflammatory reaction; however, neoplastic infiltration cannot be ruled out. Due to the slow growth rate of these tumors, they often achieve large size with minimal or no symptoms. Patient symptomatology depends primarily on the tumor location. Thus, these tumors are often discovered incidentally or may cause vague symptoms such as headache.

Schwannomas are the most common tumors of the cerebellopontine angle (80%), followed by meningiomas (10%). Other cerebellopontine angle solid lesions include ependymoma, dermoid, epidermoid, and metastatic deposits.

SUGGESTED READING

Osborn AG. *Diagnostic neuroradiology.* St. Louis: Mosby–Year Book, 1994:186, 288, 309–311.

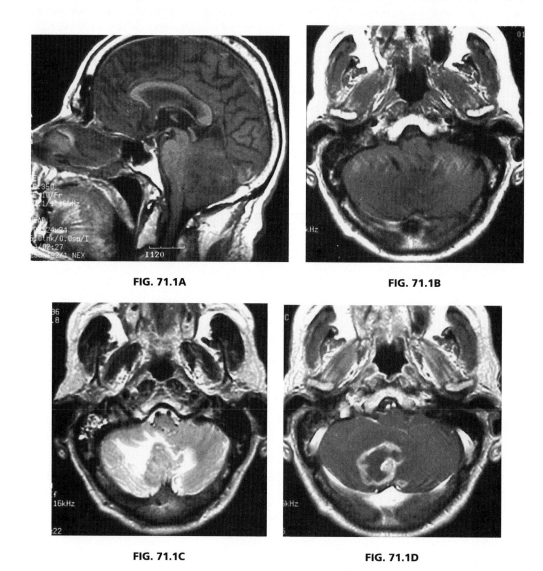

FIG. 71.1A

FIG. 71.1B

FIG. 71.1C

FIG. 71.1D

CLINICAL HISTORY

A 77-year-old man with prostate carcinoma and myesthenia gravis being treated with steroids. Patient presents with ataxia.

FINDINGS

Sagittal and axial T1-weighted acquisition (Fig. 71.1A and B) shows a large, deep hypointense mass with associated edema in the right cerebellar hemisphere. Note slight inferior displacement of the cerebellar tonsils on the sagittal acquisition. Axial T2-weighted acquisition (Fig. 71.1C) shows the mass is intermediate signal with significant perifocal edema. On postcontrast T1-weighted acquisition (Fig. 71.1D), peripheral nodular enhancement is seen. Note mass effect on the fourth ventricle with mild obstructive hydrocephalus.

DIAGNOSIS

Lymphoma.

DISCUSSION

Primary central nervous system (CNS) lymphoma is an uncommon but increasingly diagnosed tumor, which occurs in two different patient populations: immunologically normal patients and immunocompromised patients. The site of origin is unknown since the CNS contains no endogenous lymphoid tissue or lymphatic circulation. Lymphoma in the immunologically normal population typically presents in the sixth decade while acquired immunodeficiency syndrome–related disease presents in the fourth decade.

Pathologically, CNS lymphoma can be a circumscribed or a poorly defined infiltrating tumor. It can extend along the perivascular (Virchow-Robin) spaces and infiltrate blood vessel walls. Histologically, one sees small densely packed neoplastic lymphocytes concentrated in a perivascular pattern.

The classic imaging finding is a large rounded mass lesion involving the deep gray matter, periventricular regions, and/or corpus callosum. Lymphoma is isodense to hyperdense on CT due to its dense cellularity, with homogeneous enhancement. Most lesions are isointense to hypointense to gray matter on T1-weighted images. Lesions are characteristically isointense to slightly hypointense on T2-weighted images, again related to dense cellularity and high nuclear cytoplasmic ratio. Hyperintense lesions can, however, be seen in more necrotic lesions. Seventy-five percent of lesions are in contact with the ependyma, meninges, or both, and most lesions (75% to 85%) are supratentorial. There is usually very little edema relative to lesion size. In approximately 50% of cases, the lesions are multiple. There is typically strong homogeneous enhancement in the immunocompetent population (see Volume 2, Case 47). If there is enhancement along the perivascular spaces, lymphoma should be the number one diagnostic consideration, followed by sarcoidosis (see Cases 49 and 79). Calcification and hemorrhage are uncommon in CNS lymphoma in an immunologically normal patient.

In immunocompromised patients with primary CNS lymphoma, signal characteristics are more heterogeneous and the lesions are typically ring enhancing because of the higher degree of necrosis in this population (nicely demonstrated in this case). Hemorrhagic lesions are more common and there is a higher incidence of multifocal disease. Perifocal edema is also reported to be more significant in this population.

Primary CNS lymphoma may present as a diffusely infiltrative lesion without discrete mass lesion. There is involvement of both deep gray matter nuclei and white matter tracts. When there is a "butterfly" pattern of spread across the corpus callosum, discrimination from gliomatosis cerebri is not possible (see Volume 2, Case 59).

In the immunocompromised population, the multifocal enhancing lesions seen in CNS lymphoma are difficult, if not impossible, to distinguished from common opportunistic CNS infections, specifically toxoplasmosis. Differentiation based on imaging criteria is challenging and generally not reliable. The literature highlights some helpful, although not foolproof, imaging clues. A solitary lesion in an immunocompromised patient is more likely to be lymphoma and should carry a lower threshold for biopsy. Toxoplasmosis can, however, present as a solitary lesion (28% to 39%). In general, the average lesion size is larger in lymphoma. Hyperattenuation on noncontrast CT and the presence of subependymal spread of tumor have been reported as the most reliable features in the diagnosis of primary CNS lymphoma, as opposed to toxoplasmosis in the immunocompromised patient. Thallium radionuclide scanning is very helpful, being positive in lymphoma but not toxoplasmosis.

Differential diagnosis in the immunocompetent population with primary CNS lymphoma includes glioma, metastasis, and sarcoid. On noncontrast CT, the hyperdense lesions can mimic vascular lesions, such as cavernous hemangiomas or arteriovenous malformation.

Primary CNS lymphomas are highly radiosensitive tumors. Most cases regress completely following radiotherapy. Recurrent or progressive disease is common and usually occurs within 1 year. Overall prognosis is poor with a median survival of 13.5 months after diagnosis.

In contradistinction to primary CNS lymphoma, metastasis to the CNS from systemic lymphoma (or secondary CNS lymphoma) usually manifests as dural or leptomeningeal disease. There may or may not be involvement of the underlying parenchyma.

SUGGESTED READING

Baladrishnan J, Becker PS, Kumar AJ, et al. Acquired immunodeficiency syndrome: correlation of radiologic and pathologic findings in the brain. *Radiographics* 1990;10:201–215.

Ciricillo SF, Rosenblum ML. Use of CT and MR imaging to distinguish intracranial lesions and to define the need for biopsy in AIDS patients. *J Neurosurg* 1990;73:720–724.

Dina TS. Primary central nervous system lymphoma versus toxoplasmosis in AIDS. *Radiology* 1991;179:823–828.

Johnson BA, Fram EK, Johnson PC, et al. The variable appearance of primary lymphoma of the central nervous system: comparison with histopathologic features. *AJNR* 1997;18:563–572.

Osborn AG. Meningiomas and other nonglial neoplasms. In: *Diagnostic neuroradiology*, 1st ed. St. Louis: Mosby, 1994:620–622.

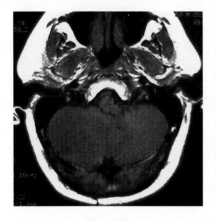

FIG. 72.1A

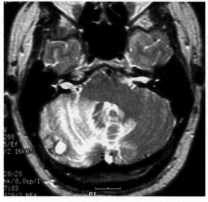

FIG. 72.1B

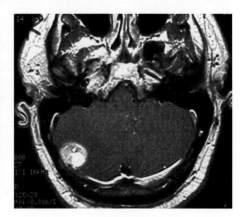

FIG. 72.1C

CLINICAL HISTORY

A 50-year-old man with ataxia.

FINDINGS

Axial T1-weighted acquisition (Fig. 72.1A) shows a small, well-circumscribed 1 to 2 cm focus of low intensity within the cortex and subcortical white matter of the right cerebellar hemisphere. There is surrounding hypointensity consistent with edema as well as mass effect upon the right lateral aspect of the fourth ventricle. There is no hydrocephalus. Axial T2-weighted acquisition (Fig. 72.1B) shows the lesion to be heterogeneous in signal with significant perifocal edema. Note serpentine regions of signal void along the surface of the cerebellar hemisphere consistent with tumor vascularity. Postcontrast acquisition (Fig. 72.1C) shows a heterogeneously enhancing well-defined mass along the pial surface of the right cerebellar hemisphere.

DIAGNOSIS

Cerebellar hemangioblastoma.

DISCUSSION

Hemangioblastoma is the most common primary tumor to occur below the tentorium in the adult population. It is a benign tumor that is easily cured with surgical excision. Most hemangioblastomas occur in the cerebellar hemispheres. Other less common locations include the spinal cord, medulla and cerebrum in decreasing order of frequency. They usually occur in adult males (30 to 65 years of age). The most common presenting symptoms are headache, ataxia, nausea, vomiting, and vertigo. Interestingly, polycythemia vera can be associated with hemangioblastoma due to the production of erythropoietin. Spinal hemangioblastoma can present with subarachnoid hemorrhage.

Hemangioblastomas typically occur sporadically (80%). Approximately, 20% of hemangioblastomas are associated with von Hippel-Lindau (VHL) syndrome. VHL syndrome is an autosomal dominant inherited disease with multiple systemic manifestations, including multiple hemangioblastomas (cerebellum, brainstem, and spinal cord), renal, pancreatic and hepatic cysts, renal cell carcinoma, pheochromocytoma, and polycythemia vera.

The typical imaging findings of hemangioblastoma are a cystic mass with a solid mural nodule, which is highly vascular and is associated with serpentine signal void related to feeding vessels. The mural nodule demonstrates striking enhancement. The cyst and its walls do not enhance. Forty percent of hemangioblastomas are purely solid with no identifiable cystic component. These lesions are typically isointense on T1-weighted images and hyperintense on T2-weighted images with intense enhancement following contrast. Purely cystic hemangioblastomas can also occur but are much less common. Hemangioblastomas characteristically abut the pial surface of the brain. Intratumoral hemorrhage is common. Peritumoral edema and mass effect are minimal unless the lesion has hemorrhaged. Most tumors are solitary, however, multiple lesions do occur (5%). Thirty percent to sixty percent are multiple in VHL.

Differential diagnosis for a vascular posterior fossa mass includes pilocytic astrocytoma, vascular malformation, and metastatic disease.

SUGGESTED READING

Hasso AN, Bell SA, Tadmor R. Intracranial vascular tumors. *Neuroimaging Clin North Am* 1994;4(4):849–870.

Ho VB, Smirniotopoulos JG, Murphy FM, et al. Radiologic-pathologic correlation: hemangioblastoma. *AJNR* 1992;13(5):1,343–1,352.

Lee SR, Sanches J, Mark AS, et al. Posterior fossa hemangioblastoma: MR imaging. *Radiology* 1989;171(2):463–468.

Osborn AG. Meningiomas and other nonglial neoplasms. In: *Diagnostic neuroradiology,* 1st ed. St. Louis: Mosby, 1994:605–607.

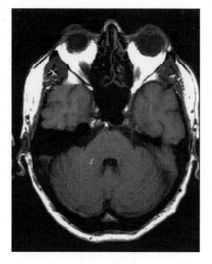

FIG. 73.1A

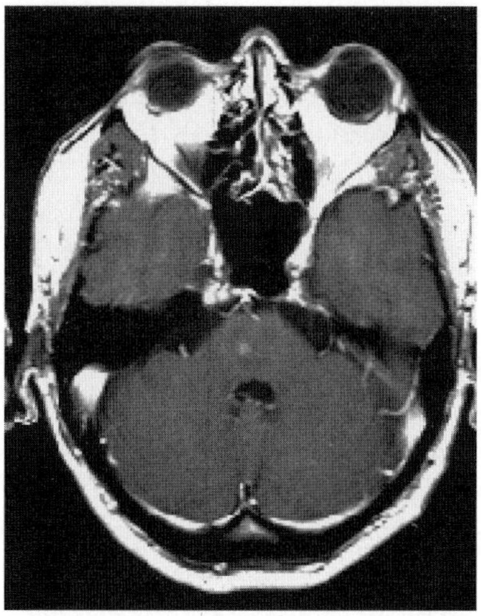

FIG. 73.1B

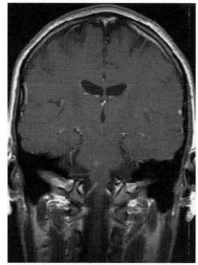

FIG. 73.1C

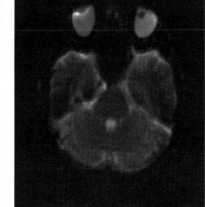

FIG. 73.1D

CLINICAL HISTORY

Headache.

FINDINGS

A 5 mm area of high signal intensity is evident within the lower right pons on the gadolinium-enhanced T1-weighted images (Fig. 73.1B and C), which is not evident on the precontrast T1-weighted image (Fig. 73.1A) or the T2-weighted EPI image (Fig. 73.1D). *Submitted by Elizabeth Vogler, M.D., Peter Brotchie, M.B.B.S., Ph.D., and William G. Bradley, M.D., Ph.D., F.A.C.R., Senior Editor, Long Beach Memorial Medical Center, Long Beach, California.*

DIAGNOSIS

Capillary telangiectasia.

DISCUSSION

Capillary telangiectasias are common lesions. They are usually clinically silent and are often found at autopsy. They are the second most common vascular malformation after venous angiomas. They can occur anywhere in the brain or spinal cord but have a predilection for the pons. Multiple lesions are common and they often coexist with other vascular malformations, particularly cavernous angiomas. Capillary telangiectasias consist of nests of dilated thin-walled capillaries, lacking smooth muscle and elastic fibers, interposed between normal brain parenchyma. There may be associated gliosis in the surrounding brain or hemosiderin staining from previous hemorrhage. Capillary telangiectasias can be associated with Rendu-Osler-Weber (hereditary hemorrhagic telangiectasia), although true arteriovenous malformations are more commonly found in this syndrome.

Capillary telangiectasias are usually seen as poorly defined foci of increased signal intensity on gadolinium-enhanced MRI. In addition, there may be multiple punctate foci of hypointensity on T2-weighted and gradient echo images, if hemorrhage has occurred. CT scan is typically normal but may demonstrate faint areas of increased density following contrast administration. Capillary telangiectasias are usually occult on cerebral angiography, although a faint vascular stain may be demonstrated.

SUGGESTED READING

Osborn AG. *Diagnostic neuroradiology.* St. Louis: Mosby–Year Book, 1994;186, 288, 309–311.

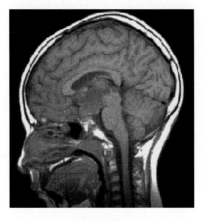

FIG. 74.1A

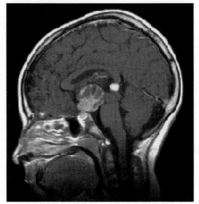

FIG. 74.1B

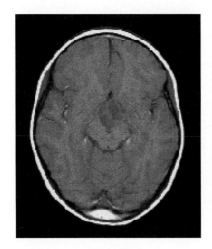

FIG. 74.1C

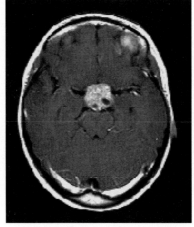

FIG. 74.1D

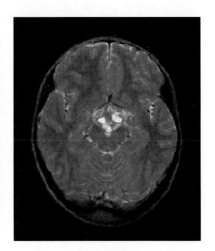

FIG. 74.1E

CLINICAL HISTORY

A 15-year-old boy with persistent headache and visual complaints.

FINDINGS

Sagittal and axial MRI demonstrates a large suprasellar mass and a smaller pineal mass, both of predominately low signal on T1-weighted images with marked enhancement (Fig. 74.1A–D). The T2-weighted image reveals heterogeneous signal intensity of the lesion (Fig. 74.1E) suggesting necrosis. *Submitted by Peter Brotchie, M.B.B.S., Ph.D., Sattam Lingawi, M.B., Ch.B., F.R.C.P.C., and William G. Bradley, M.D., Ph.D., F.A.C.R., Senior Editor, Long Beach Memorial Medical Center, Long Beach, California.*

DIAGNOSIS

Pineal germinoma with suprasellar metastasis.

DISCUSSION

Tumors of the pineal region can be divided according to the cell of origin into four categories: (i) tumors of pineal cell origin (pineoblastoma and pineocytoma), (ii) tumors of germ cell origin (germinoma, mature/immature teratoma, teratocarcinoma, embryonal carcinoma, choriocarcinoma, yolk sac tumor, and mixed germ cell tumors), (iii) tumors of other origin (glial tumors, hemangiopericytoma, and meningioma), and (iv) cysts.

α-fetoprotein (AFP) is produced by the yolk sac in the early stages of development, and human chorionic gonadotropin (HCG) is synthesized by the choroidal epithelium. Yolk sac tumors produce AFP while choriocarcinomas produce HCG. Embryonal carcinomas produce both AFP and HCG and have the potential to dedifferentiate into other germ cell tumors.

The most common pineal region tumor is the germinoma. They most commonly occur in the pineal region; however, the suprasellar location is not unusual. These tumors are highly radiosensitive and generally have a good prognosis.

There are no definite radiological findings that differentiate one cell type from another. They usually demonstrate T1 isointensity and T2 hyperintensity or hypointensity (in comparison to brain parenchyma) on MRI. The hypointensity on the long TE sequences is thought to be due to calcification (20% to 40% of cases) and a high nuclear-to-cytoplasmic ratio. The hyperintensity represents cyst formation. Gadolinium-enhanced images usually reveal an intense heterogeneous pattern of enhancement.

Extension of pineal tumors can occur through one of three pathways: (i) seeding via the cerebrospinal fluid, (ii) via direct continuity, and (iii) via the bloodstream.

SUGGESTED READING

Chang T, Teng M, Guo W, et al. CT of pineal tumors and intracranial germ cell tumors. *AJNR* 1989;153:1239–1244.

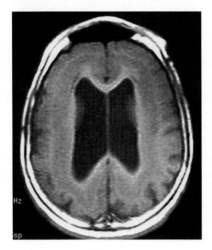

FIG. 75.1A

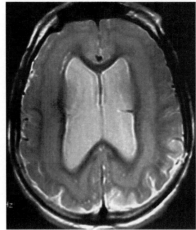

FIG. 75.1B

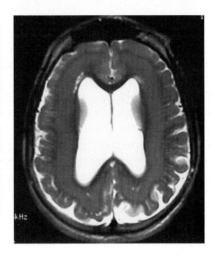

FIG. 75.1C

CLINICAL HISTORY

An 11-year-old girl with history of seizures.

FINDINGS

Axial T1-weighted (Fig. 75.1A), proton density (Fig. 75.1B), and T2-weighted (Fig. 75.1C) images demonstrate prominence of the lateral ventricles. There is a thick band of abnormal signal within the central white matter of both cerebral hemispheres. The signal abnormality is bilateral and symmetric and follows gray matter signal on all pulse sequences.

DIAGNOSIS

Band heterotopia.

DISCUSSION

Gray matter heterotopia is one entity in a spectrum of congenital abnormalities known as the "neuronal migrational disorders" (NMDs). NMDs accounted for 4.3% of all epilepsy patients referred for MRI in one study. Although they are congenital disorders, the onset of seizures is surprisingly late, often after 10 years of age. It is uncertain if heterotopic gray matter is the actual cause of seizures or if it is a marker of an abnormal process that results in seizure activity.

NMDs range from gray matter heterotopias to sulcation anomalies, depending on the time and extent of migration arrest. Heterotopia represents the earliest migrational arrest, in which a collection of normal gray matter is found in an abnormal location. Nodular heterotopia is a focus or foci of gray matter that never migrates and is usually found in the subependymal region. Laminar or band heterotopia occurs when there is diffuse arrest of neuronal migration resulting in a layer of ectopic gray matter between the ventricles and cortex. Occasionally, heterotopia presents as a large mass of dysplastic gray matter involving part or all of a cerebral hemisphere. Heterotopia may be an isolated finding or associated with other sulcation anomalies (e.g., pachygyria or polymicrogyria) and dysplasias (e.g., corpus callosum).

Because MRI is superior to CT in differentiating gray and white matter, it is the modality of choice in imaging NMDs. Nodular heterotopia (see Case 28) appears as multiple confluent subependymal masses, which are identical in signal intensity to gray matter on all pulse sequences. There is no enhancement following contrast. The characteristic signal intensity helps to differentiate this entity from the subependymal nodules seen in tuberous sclerosis, which demonstrate high signal on T2-weighted acquisition and can enhance (see Case 46). Band heterotopia features a thick symmetric band of gray matter within the centrum semiovale, interposed between the ventricles and cortex. There is typically a thin layer of residual normal white matter between the heterotopic gray matter and normal overlying cortex.

This case illustrates the band-type or laminar-type gray matter heterotopia.

SUGGESTED READING

Barkovich AJ, Kjos BO. Gray matter heterotopia: MR characteristics and correlation with developmental and neurologic manifestations. *Radiology* 1992;182(2):493–499.

Brodtkorb E, Nilsen G, Smevik O, et al. Epilepsy and abnormalities of neuronal migration: MRI and clinical aspects. *Acta Neurol Scand* 1992;86:24–32.

Canapicchi R, Padolecchia R, Puglioli M, et al. Heterotopic gray matter. Neuroradiological aspects and clinical correlation. *J Neuroradiol* 1990;17(4):277–287.

Hayden SA, Davis KA, Stears JC, et al. MR imaging of heterotopic gray matter. *JCAT* 1987;11(5):878–879.

Smith AS, Weinstein MA, Quencer RM, et al. Association of heterotopic gray matter with seizures: MR imaging. Work in progress. *Radiology* 1988;168(1):195–198.

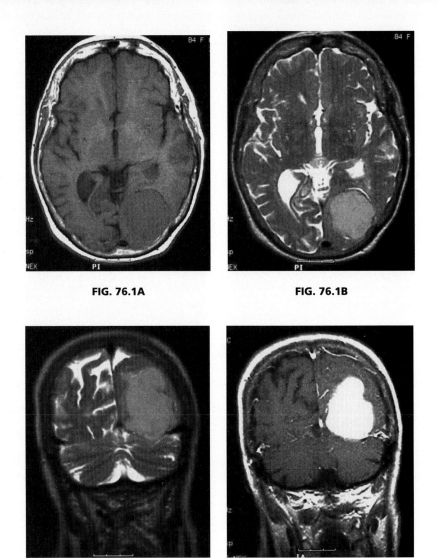

FIG. 76.1A

FIG. 76.1B

FIG. 76.1C

FIG. 76.1D

CLINICAL HISTORY

An 84-year-old woman with visual disturbance.

FINDINGS

Axial T1-weighted acquisition (Fig. 76.1A) shows a large, rounded, well-defined isointense mass within the left occipital lobe. There is mass effect upon the atrium of the left lateral ventricle, as well as effacement of cortical sulci. Axial and coronal T2-weighted acquisitions (Fig. 76.1B and C) demonstrate the mass to be isointense to slightly hyperintense in signal. There is very little perilesional edema for a lesion of this size. The coronal acquisition demonstrates a broad base of attachment along the left leaf of the tentorium. Postcontrast images (Fig. 76.1D) demonstrate well-defined, homogenous enhancement. There is extension of tumor below the tentorium. The dural venous sinuses are patent.

DIAGNOSIS

Meningioma.

DISCUSSION

Meningiomas are the most common primary nonglial intracranial tumor. They are most commonly found in middle-aged and older people. There is a female predominance of 2:1 in the adult population. Meningiomas are rare in the pediatric population and when present are frequently associated with neurofibromatosis. The possibility of neurofibromatosis should be considered in any patient with multiple meningiomas. Meningiomas often coexist in patients with breast carcinoma. They have also been seen to arise in patients several years after "radiation-induced" meningioma.

Meningiomas arise from the meninges or cell rests of meningeal derivation. They have a predilection for areas associated with arachnoid granulations and are most often found along the convexity attached to the sagittal sinus. Other favorite areas include the dura adjacent to the anterior sylvian fissure, the sphenoid wing, tuberculum sellae, perisellar region, and olfactory grooves. In the posterior fossa, they tend to arise along the petrous bone in the cerebellopontine angle, the clivus, along the tentorial leaf, and at the free edge of the tentorium. Meningiomas usually have a broad base of dural attachment but can occasionally arise without dural attachment within the sylvian fissure or ventricles. The lateral ventricle is the most commonly involved, followed by the third and fourth ventricles.

The first and most important step in the diagnosis of meningioma is to determine whether the tumor is extraaxial. There are several criteria to help make this decision. A broad-based dural attachment is strongly suggestive but not definitive. Bony hyperostosis and/or calvarial invasion are highly specific for extraaxial origin. The other highly specific sign is the visualization of pial vascular structures, cerebrospinal fluid (CSF) clefts, and dural margins between the tumor and cerebral cortex. Pial blood vessel interfaces appear as punctate and curvilinear signal voids on all pulse sequences at the junction of the tumor with underlying brain. The vascular structures may be arteries or veins. About 80% of meningiomas will demonstrate a vascular margin at the interface with the brain. Eighty percent of meningiomas will also demonstrate a CSF cleft between the tumor and underlying brain parenchyma. The dural margin interface is seen primarily in meningiomas of the cavernous sinus. It appears as a low-intensity rim on all pulse sequences separating the tumor from the adjacent temporal lobe (see Volume 2, Case 34). Often, however, the tumor can be seen to invade directly through the dura and abut the adjacent brain. Meningiomas along the falx and tentorium, as in this case, can also invade through the dura to its opposite side. It is important to note that intraaxial tumors almost never invade the dura unless there has been previous surgery. Metastases can occasionally grow exophytically from brain parenchyma and invade dura, however, there will be no tumor-brain interface.

Another valuable tool in determining whether a mass is extraaxial is the buckling of the cortical gyri subjacent to the extraaxial mass into an "onionskin-like" configuration beginning at the margin of the tumor. This sign is better seen on MRI and with large meningiomas.

On unenhanced CT, meningiomas are usually slightly hyperdense. The tumor is calcified in approximately 20% of cases. Rarely, meningiomas show cystic, osteoblastic, chondromatous, or fatty degeneration. On MRI, the typical signal characteristics consist of isointense to slightly hypointense signal relative to gray matter on T1-weighted images and range from hypointense to hyperintense signal relative to gray matter on T2-weighted images. There is characteristically intense homogenous enhancement of meningiomas. Occasionally, they have necrotic centers, which may not enhance. The dural tail, a crescentic tail of enhancement at the tumor-dura interface, is typically seen with meningioma, although it is not specific. Dural metastases and occasionally schwannomas can show this uncommonly. The degree of parenchymal edema within subjacent brain is variable, the slow growth of the tumor often produces brain atrophy, thus, little mass effect may be seen with large lesions. Rarely, meningiomas invade underlying brain parenchyma.

Meningioma can also grow in an "en plaque" fashion, appearing as a region of diffuse dural thickening. Differentiation from dural metastasis, lymphoma, and sarcoidosis can be difficult.

Meningiomas may encase and narrow adjacent vessels, most notably when they occur in the parasellar region (see Volume 2, Case 34). Adjacent dural venous sinuses can be invaded and/or occluded (see Volume 2, Case 21). Bony changes associated with meningiomas may be hyperostotic or osteolytic in nature. Meningioma can even invade through the calvarium and present as a scalp mass (see Volume 2, Case 21). Sphenoid or ethmoid sinus expansion can be seen with adjacent meningioma.

Complete surgical excision is the treatment of choice. A recent study described more frequent recurrence of lobulated or "mushrooming" meningiomas as compared to rounded tumors. These tumors, therefore, require a more aggressive surgical approach with wider surgical margins. Important preoperative imaging issues for meningioma include invasion of underlying parenchyma, invasion of the cavernous sinus, compression or invasion of the dural venous sinuses, and/or the presence of vascular encasement.

SUGGESTED READING

Elster AD, Challa VR, Gilbert TH, et al. Meningioma: MR and histopathological features. *Radiology* 1989;170:857–862.

Wasenko JJ, Hochhauser L, Stopa EG, et al. Cystic meningioma: MR characteristics and surgical correlation. *AJNR* 1994;15(10):1,959–1,965.

Nakasu S, Nakasu Y, Nakajima M, et al. Preoperative identification of meningiomas that are highly likely to recur. *J Neurosurg* 1999;90(3):455–462.

Osborn AG. Meningiomas and other nonglial neoplasms. In: *Diagnostic neuroradiology,* 1st ed. St.Louis: Mosby, 1994:584–601.

Goldsher D, Litt AW, Pinto RS, et al. Dural "tail" associated with meningiomas on Gd-DTPA-enhanced MR images: characteristics, differential diagnostic value, and possible implications for treatment. *Radiology* 1990;176:447–450.

Goldberg HI, Lavi E, Atlas SW. Extra-axial brain tumors. In: Atlas SW, ed. *Magnetic resonance imaging of the brain and spine,* 2nd ed. Philadelphia: Lippincott–Raven Publishers, 1996:424–446.

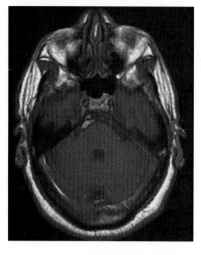

FIG. 77.1A

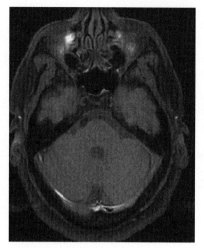

FIG. 77.1B

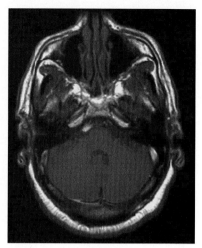

FIG. 77.1C

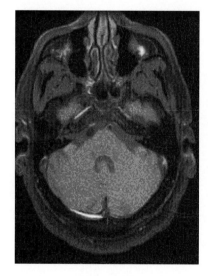

FIG. 77.1D

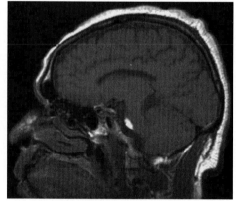

FIG. 77.1E

CLINICAL HISTORY

A 48-year-old man with headaches.

FINDINGS

A small hyperintense lesion is evident in the anterior right cerebellopontine angle on the T1-weighted images (Fig. 77.1A, C, E). The lesion becomes hypointense with fat suppression (Fig. 77.1B and D). *Submitted by Kathleen Flores, M.D., Sattam Lingawi, M.B., Ch.B., F.R.C.P.C., Peter Brotchie, M.B.B.S., Ph.D., and William G. Bradley, M.D., Ph.D., F.A.C.R., Senior Editor, Long Beach Memorial Medical Center, Long Beach, California.*

DIAGNOSIS

Intracranial lipoma.

DISCUSSION

Intracranial lipomas are histologically benign and usually incidental MRI findings. With the current liberal use of MRI, these are becoming identified more frequently in various intracranial compartments. They occur most commonly in the trigonal choroid plexus, cerebral convexity, middle and posterior cranial fossae, and pericallosal and quadrigeminal cistern regions. They are considered congenital hamartomatous malformations derived from meninx primitiva. They have been associated with varying degrees of intracranial malformations, the most common of which is dysgenesis of the corpus callosum. In the vast majority of cases in which intracranial lipomas are discovered, they are not related to the patient's neurological symptoms.

The MRI appearance of lipomas is characteristic. They are hyperintense on T1-weighted images and dark on conventional T2-weighted images. They have chemical shift artifact, best seen on proton density–weighted images. On T1-weighted images, the bright signal can be nulled using spectroscopic fat saturation at high field or short TI inversion recovery (STIR) at any field. (Although they are hypointense on T2-weighted conventional spin echo images, on fast spin echo images, they remain hyperintense due to decoupling of the J-coupled spin system by a Carr-Purcell-Meiboom-Gill echo train.)

SUGGESTED READING

Bakshi R, Shaikh Z, Kamran S, et al. MRI findings in 32 consecutive lipomas using conventional and advanced sequences. *J Neuroimaging* 1999;9:134–140.

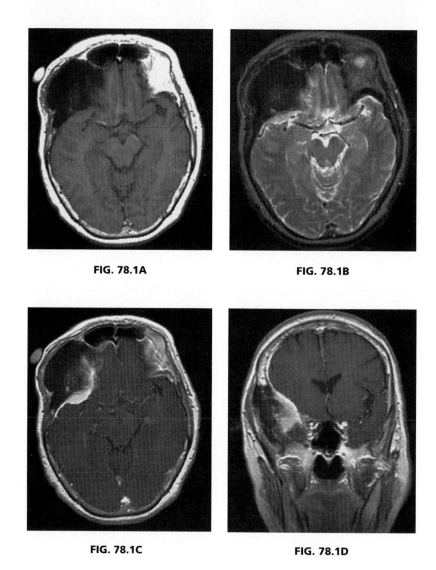

FIG. 78.1A **FIG. 78.1B**

FIG. 78.1C **FIG. 78.1D**

CLINICAL HISTORY

A 62-year-old woman with history of a slow-growing lump on her head.

FINDINGS

There is an intraosseous right frontal mass, which is dark on both T1-weighted and T2-weighted sequences (Fig. 78.1A and B). Although the bony portion does not enhance, the intraosseous component does in an "en plaque" configuration (Fig. 78.1C and D). *Submitted by Stephanie Chiu, M.D., Sattam Lingawi, M.B., Ch.B., F.R.C.P.C., Peter Brotchie, M.B.B.S., Ph.D., and William G. Bradley, M.D., Ph.D., F.A.C.R., Senior Editor, Long Beach Memorial Medical Center, Long Beach, California.*

DIAGNOSIS

Intraosseous meningioma.

DISCUSSION

Intraosseous meningiomas are rare benign tumors. They are believed to arise from arachnoidal rests that were either congenitally trapped or traumatically driven into the extradural space. Thus, it is not surprising that they most commonly occur near calvarial sutures and fracture lines. These lesions usually incite intense sclerotic (osteoblastic) reaction secondary to infiltration of tumor cells into haversian canals; however, osteolytic meningiomas have also been reported. The tumor often infiltrates all the way through the calvarial bones resulting in a subcutaneous component. The expansion due to hyperostosis may lead to a noticeable bump (as in this case). These changes are easily seen on both CT and MRI. Enhanced images in both modalities help to outline the extraosseous component of the meningioma.

The differential diagnosis includes osteoma, Paget disease, osteomyelitis, fibrous dysplasia, hemangioma, and calvarial sarcoma.

SUGGESTED READING

Lee H, Prager J, Hahn Y, et al. Intraosseous meningioma: CT and MRI appearance. *JCAT* 1992;16(6):1,000–1,001.

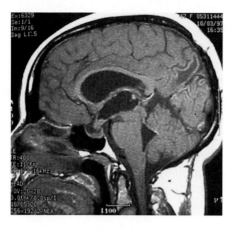

FIG. 79.1A

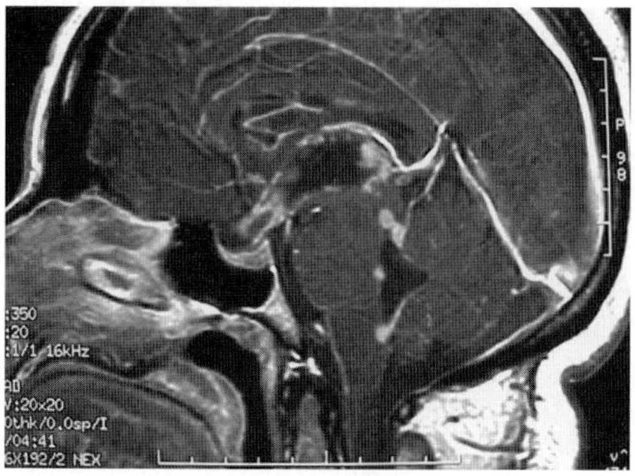

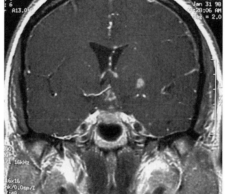

FIG. 79.1B

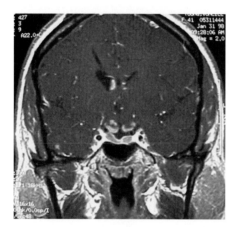

FIG. 79.1C

FIG. 79.1D

CLINICAL HISTORY

A 41-year-old woman with headache and cranial nerve neuropathy.

FINDINGS

Sagittal and coronal precontrast and postcontrast (Fig. 79.1A–D) T1-weighted images demonstrate marked nodular enhancement along the ependymal surface of the lateral third and fourth ventricles, as well as within the basal cisterns with extension along the infundibulum and optic nerves. There are several focal rounded regions of parenchymal enhancement. A right-sided ventricular drain is present.

DIAGNOSIS

Central nervous system (CNS) sarcoidosis.

DISCUSSION

Sarcoidosis is a systemic granulomatous disease of unknown etiology that most commonly occurs in the third and fourth decades. Neurological manifestations of sarcoidosis occur in only 5% of patients with the disease. Neurosarcoidosis usually develops in patients with known systemic disease or rarely as the initial manifestation. Sarcoid granulomas have been found in the CNS in up to 14% of cases at autopsy in patients with known disease. The CNS manifestations include cranial neuropathies, meningitis, hydrocephalus, and/or focal neurological deficit related to parenchymal mass lesion. Hypothalamic dysfunction is particularly common because of the propensity of sarcoid granulomas to involve the basal cisterns.

There are several different imaging manifestations of neurosarcoidosis. The most common pattern of disease is a diffuse leptomeningitis, with particular involvement of the basal cisterns, hypothalamus, pituitary stalk, optic nerves, and chiasm (as seen in this case). Focal intrasellar and suprasellar mass lesions have also been described. Neurosarcoidosis can also present as single or multiple parenchymal mass lesions. There is a predilection for the periventricular white matter and ventricular ependyma. With leptomeningeal disease, the subjacent brain parenchyma can be involved due to direct infiltration of the brain via the perivascular spaces. When there is perivascular space involvement, there can also be invasion and thrombosis of perforating blood vessels, producing a granulomatous angiitis of the CNS. Dural-based mass lesions are also a common manifestation of neurosarcoidosis.

On T1-weighted images, leptomeningeal disease usually presents as an isointense thick rind of granulomatous tissue within the subarachnoid space, extending along the surface of the brain. There may or may not be extension into the cortical sulci. Findings may be focal or diffuse. On T2-weighted acquisition, the granulomatous process is usually hypointense due to its dense cellular nature. Parenchymal edema may be present due to direct infiltration of brain parenchyma and/or ischemic change related to small vessel vasculitis. Parenchymal mass lesions usually homogeneously enhance following contrast and can be difficult to distinguish from primary CNS neoplasm. With perivascular extension of disease, linear foci of parenchymal enhancement (along the Virchow-Robin spaces) can be identified. This finding, when present, has been described as a characteristic finding in neurosarcoidosis and is highly suggestive of the disease. Lymphoma is the other entity that should be considered when a linear enhancement pattern is identified. Dural-based neurosarcoidosis is virtually indistinguishable from "en plaque" meningioma or dural lymphoma. Multifocal periventricular disease can mimic multiple sclerosis and other demyelinating disease.

In the setting of diffuse nodular leptomeningitis, as seen in this case, the differential diagnosis should include neurosarcoidosis, carcinomatous, or infectious meningitis (tuberculosis, fungal, less commonly bacterial), and lymphoma.

SUGGESTED READING

Goldberg HI, Lavi E, Atlas SW. Extra-axial brain tumors. In: *Magnetic resonance imaging of the brain and spine,* 2nd ed. Philadelphia: Lippincott–Raven Publishers, 1996:448–449.

Handler MS, Johnson LM, Dick AR, et al. Neurosarcoidosis with unusual MRI findings. *Neuroradiology* 1993;35(2):146–148.

Hayes WS, Sherman JL, Stern BJ, et al. MR and CT evaluation of intracranial sarcoidosis. *AJNR* 1987;8:841–847.

Lexa FJ, Grossman RI. MR of sarcoidosis in the head and spine: spectrum of manifestations and radiographic response to steroid therapy. *AJNR* 1994;15(5):973–982.

Lipper MH, Goldstein JM. Neurosarcoidosis mimicking a cerebellar pontine angle meningioma. *AJR* 1998;171(1):275–276.

Sherman JL, Stern BJ. Sarcoidosis of the CNS: comparison of unenhanced and enhanced MR images. *AJNR* 1990;11:915–923.

Smith AS, Meisler DM, Weinstein MA, et al. High-signal lesions in patients with sarcoidosis: neurosarcoidosis or multiple sclerosis? *AJR* 1989;153(1):147–152.

Zouaoui A, Maillard JC, Dormont D, et al. MRI in neurosarcoidosis. *J Neuroradiol* 1992;19(4):271–284.

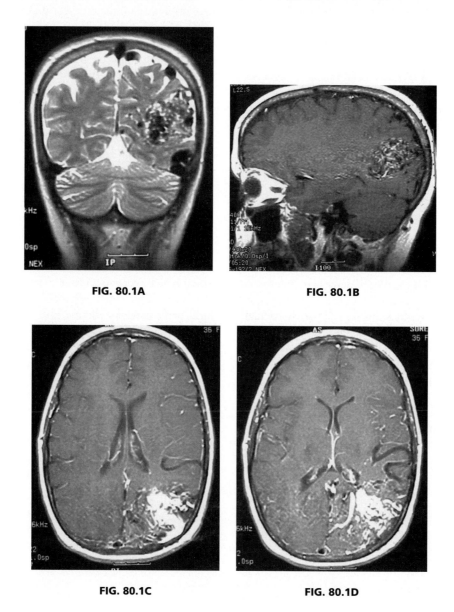

FIG. 80.1A

FIG. 80.1B

FIG. 80.1C

FIG. 80.1D

CLINICAL HISTORY

A 36-year-old woman with headache and transient right-sided weakness.

FINDINGS

There is a large tangle of vessels eliciting signal void within the left parietooccipital lobe seen on the coronal T2-weighted acquisition (Fig. 80.1A). Note the enlargement of the cortical veins and transverse and superior sagittal sinus. There are patchy hyperintense foci on the T2-weighted image adjacent to the regions of signal void consistent with regions of gliosis. Sagittal noncontrast T1-weighted acquisi-

tion (Fig. 80.1B) shows several foci of high signal, most likely related to regions of slow flow or hemorrhage. Note pulsation artifact in the phase encoding direction. Following injection of contrast (Fig. 80.1C and D), enhancement of large feeding arteries and draining veins, as well as enhancement of the nidus, is seen. Vessels with high-velocity flow do not demonstrate enhancement.

DIAGNOSIS

Arterial venous malformation.

DISCUSSION

The major purpose of MRI in the evaluation of large arterial venous malformations is not just to make the diagnosis, which is easily done when the classic picture shown here is demonstrated, but also to depict any evidence of previous hemorrhage, as patient management is much more expeditious when previous hemorrhage can be documented. The presence of infarction in association with arteriovenous malformations can also occasionally be depicted as brain substance loss.

The pathologic picture of large arteriovenous malformations is typically that of brain atrophy; however, this is due to the fact that pathologists see the brain after death, with the vascular space decompressed. *In vivo,* the pulsatile expanded vascular space produces mass effect with arteriovenous malformations; however, that mass effect can be mitigated by underlying parenchymal atrophy, and thus, a balanced picture of relatively little mass effect can be seen even with very large arteriovenous malformations. Hemorrhage would be evidenced by hemosiderin staining of the brain, infarction by gliosis, and increased water content (microcystic encephalomalacia).

Associated aneurysms can occasionally be depicted with arteriovenous malformations; nevertheless, the definitive evaluation of arteriovenous malformation for purposes of management still requires conventional angiography.

SUGGESTED READING

Lemme-Plaghos L, Kucharczyk W, Brant-Zawadzki M, et al. MR imaging of angiographically occult vascular malformations. *AJR* 1986;146:1223–1228.

Meder JF, Oppenheim C, Blustajn J, et al. Cerebral arteriovenous malformations: the value of radiologic parameters in predicting response to radiosurgery. *AJNR* 1997;18:1,473–1,483.

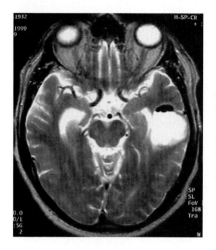

FIG. 81.1A

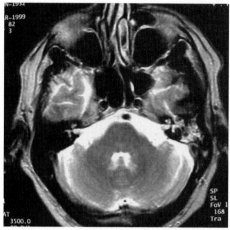

FIG. 81.1B

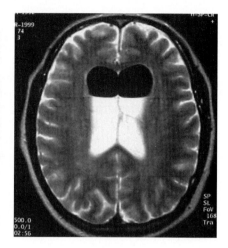

FIG. 81.1C

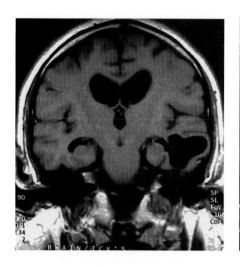

FIG. 81.1D

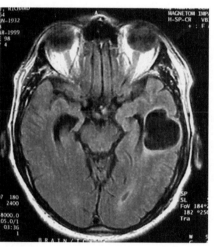

FIG. 81.1E

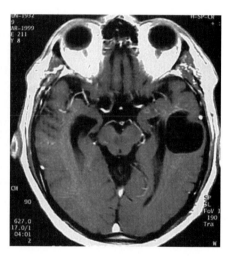

FIG. 81.1F

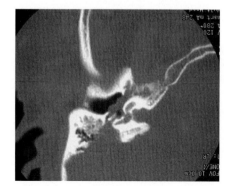

FIG. 81.1G

CLINICAL HISTORY

A 67-year-old man with history of headaches with no known trauma.

FINDINGS

Axial T2-weighted acquisitions (Fig. 81A–C) demonstrate a fluid and air filled cavity within the left temporal lobe just above the temporal ridge. This cavity measures approximately 3.5 cm. More inferiorly, there is opacification of the left mastoid air cells. Air-fluid levels are seen within the frontal horns of the lateral ventricles. The cavity abuts but does not appear to communicate with the temporal horn of the left lateral ventricle. Coronal T1-weighted acquisition (Fig. 81.1D) shows a large, well-defined, low-signal mass within the left temporal lobe. It is in contiguity with the petrous apex. Axial fluid-attenuated inversion-recovery acquisition (Fig. 81.1E) again demonstrates a well-defined hypointense mass. There is a thin peripheral rim of high signal consistent with edema and/or gliosis. Following intravenous contrast, the T1-weighted axial image (Fig. 81.1F) shows no significant enhancement.

DIAGNOSIS

Cystic cavity in the left temporal lobe with associated pneumocephalus and left otomastoiditis.

DISCUSSION

This is a very unusual case in that the patient had no history that would be consistent with cerebritis, meningitis, or abscess formation. Nonetheless, an infection must have been the cause of the lesion depicted here, particularly given the surgical finding of a dehiscence tegmen tympani with history of previous mastoid infections. There was actually herniation of brain contents into the temporal bone at surgery.

Thus, at some point, a smoldering infection must have developed in the temporal lobe overlying the temporal bone, had been handled by the patient's defense mechanisms such that a walled-off abscess occurred, and over time had become sterile. Continued communication between the air space of the mastoid antra and middle ear leads to the development of the pneumocephalus and the fluid-air–filled cavity.

Following surgery, with repair of the tegmental defect, and ventricular peritoneal shunting, the picture evolved to a simple focus of cystic encephalomalacia.

High-resolution CT scan through the left temporal bone in the coronal plane (Fig. 81.1G) shows opacification of the left middle-ear cavity with erosion of the tegmen tympani and roof of the petrous bone. Soft tissue is in contiguity with the brain parenchyma in the epitympanic region. The scutum is intact. There is opacification of the left mastoid air cells.

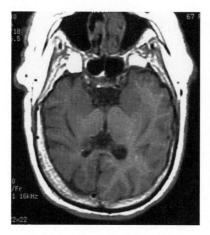

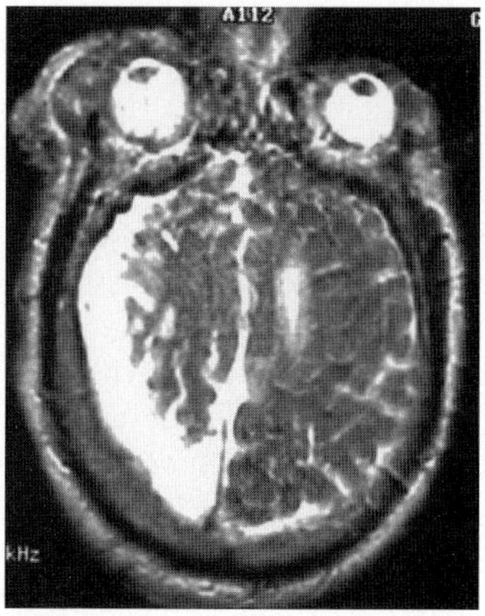

FIG. 82.1A

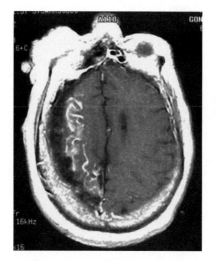

FIG. 82.1B

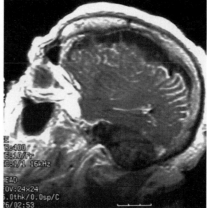

FIG. 82.1C

FIG. 82.1D

CLINICAL HISTORY

A 67-year-old woman with long-standing seizures.

FINDINGS

Axial noncontrast T1-weighted image (Fig. 82.1A) shows marked atrophy of the right cerebral hemisphere. There is thickening of the overlying calvarium, as well as enlargement of the right paranasal sinuses. Axial T2-weighted images (Fig. 82.1B) show no signal abnormality within the brain parenchyma. Following intravenous contrast (Fig. 82.1C and D), there is gyriform enhancement along the surface of the right cerebral hemisphere, as well as a markedly enlarged, enhancing choroid plexus within the right lateral ventricle. Note large lobulated soft tissue mass overlying the right cheek and orbit.

DIAGNOSIS

Sturge-Weber syndrome.

DISCUSSION

Sturge-Weber syndrome is a rare, nonhereditary neurocutaneous syndrome. Classic clinical manifestations include facial port wine nevus (usually in the V1 distribution), hemiplegia, and seizures. Buphthalmos, congenital glaucoma, mental retardation, and choroidal or scleral hemangiomas have also been described.

There are four vascular abnormalities seen in Sturge-Weber syndrome. Pial or leptomeningeal angiomatosis is the primary abnormality and is most commonly described. Absent or diminished cortical veins overlying the involved cortex, compensatory enlargement of the deep venous system, and choroid plexus enlargement (angiomatous malformation) are other associated vascular anomalies.

The classically described radiographic findings include, unilateral (occasionally bilateral) cerebral atrophy, most common posteriorly, and cortical calcification. Calcification is best seen on CT but is usually not present before the age of 2. Gradient echo sequences are sensitive in the detection of cortical calcification because of magnetic susceptibility effect. Both the cortical atrophy and calcification are the result of chronic ischemic change within cortex underlying the leptomeningeal angioma. Because of long-standing hemiatrophy, the calvarium will grow asymmetrically to maintain a symmetric outward appearance. This results in ipsilateral calvarial thickening and hypertrophy or enlargement of the ipsilateral paranasal sinuses. The constellation of findings (cerebral hemiatrophy, ipsilateral calvarial thickening, and large sinuses) is referred to as "Dyke-Davidoff-Mason syndrome."

MRI is better than CT for evaluating the extent of vascular malformation in Sturge-Weber syndrome. Cortical enhancement on postcontrast imaging (as seen in this case) is thought to represent the leptomeningeal angioma and probably disruption of the blood–brain barrier secondary to chronic cortical ischemia. There may be patchy gliosis and demyelination within the subjacent brain parenchyma. Enlargement of the ipsilateral choroid plexus and prominence of the deep venous structures are common imaging features.

SUGGESTED READING

Benedikt RA, Brown DC, Walker R, et al. Sturge-Weber syndrome: cranial MR imaging with Gd-DTPA. *AJNR* 1993;14(Mar/Apr):409–415.

Elster AD, Chen MYM. MR imaging of Sturge-Weber syndrome: role of gadopentetate dimeglumine and gradient-echo techniques. *AJNR* 1990;11(Jul/Aug):685–689.

Smirniotopoulos JG, Murphy FM. Central nervous system manifestations of the phakomatoses and other inherited syndromes. In: Atlas SW, ed. *Magnetic resonance imaging of the brain and spine,* 2nd ed. Philadelphia: Lippincott–Raven Publishers, 1996:790–794.

Wasenko JJ, Rosenbloom SA, Duchesneau PM, et al. The Sturge-Weber syndrome: comparison of MR and CT characteristics. *AJNR* 1990; 11(Jan/Feb):131–134.

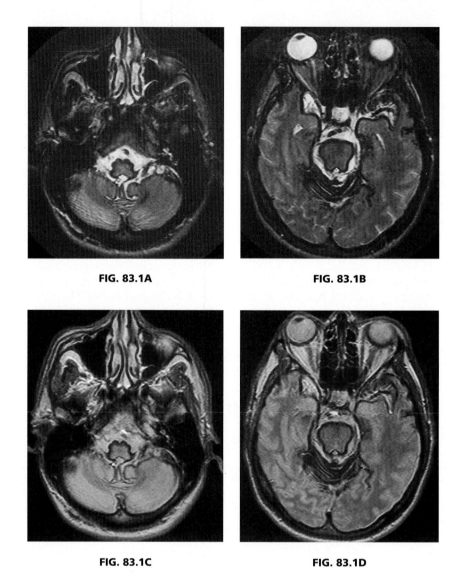

FIG. 83.1A

FIG. 83.1B

FIG. 83.1C

FIG. 83.1D

CLINICAL HISTORY

A 41-year-old man with deafness and history of several previous episodes of subarachnoid hemorrhage.

FINDINGS

The surface of the brain appears as if it were outlined in black, more pronounced on the T2-weighted images (Fig. 83.1A and B) than the proton density–weighted images (Fig. 83.1C and D). *Submitted by William G. Bradley, M.D., Ph.D., F.A.C.R., Senior Editor, Long Beach Memorial Medical Center, Long Beach, California.*

DIAGNOSIS

Superficial siderosis.

DISCUSSION

Hemosiderin, a paramagnetic breakdown product of hemoglobin, is readily detected as low signal on MRI. This is most pronounced on T2-weighted gradient echo images, less pronounced on T2-weighted conventional spin echo images (as in this case), and least pronounced on T2-weighted fast spin echo images (which tend to minimize a magnetic susceptibility effects).

Superficial siderosis represents hemosiderin deposition in the leptomeninges. The leptomeninges cover the brain and the cranial nerves. The most common presentation of superficial siderosis is deafness, although other cranial nerve palsies can also occur. While mild subarachnoid hemorrhage is generally cleared by the arachnoid villi, more protracted exposure due to oozing or repeated subarachnoid hemorrhage results in hemosiderin deposition in the pia and arachnoid.

SUGGESTED READING

Fearnley JM, Stevens JM, Rudge P. Superficial siderosis of the central nervous system. *Brain* 1995;118(4): 1,051–1,066.

Offenbacher H, Fazekas F, Schmidt R, et al. Superficial siderosis of the central nervous system: MRI findings and clinical significance. *Neuroradiology* 1996;38(Suppl 1):51–56.

Uchino A, Aibe H, Itoh H, et al. Superficial siderosis of the central nervous system. Its MRI manifestations. *Clin Imaging* 1997;21:241–245.

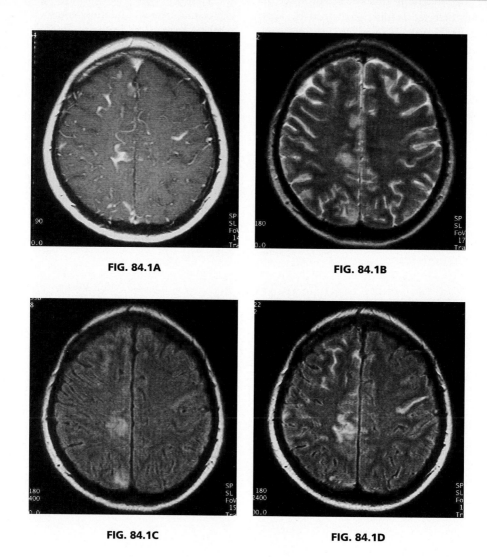

FIG. 84.1A

FIG. 84.1B

FIG. 84.1C

FIG. 84.1D

CLINICAL HISTORY

A 31-year-old man presenting with severe headache progressing to coma.

FINDINGS

Multiple areas of leptomeningeal enhancement are noted following administration of gadolinium (Fig. 84.1A). Many of these areas of enhancement show increased signal on T2-weighted (Fig. 84.1B) and fluid-attenuated inversion-recovery (FLAIR) images (Fig. 84.1C), indicating associated vasogenic edema in the brain. This is best seen on the enhanced FLAIR images (Fig. 84.1D). *Submitted by William G. Bradley, M.D., Ph.D., F.A.C.R., Senior Editor, Long Beach Memorial Medical Center, Long Beach, California.*

DIAGNOSIS

Meningitis with secondary cerebritis.

DISCUSSION

With progression of meningitis and/or more virulent organisms, the brain itself becomes infected, leading to cerebritis. This is best seen on T2-weighted and FLAIR images. (FLAIR images are also very T2-weighted except they have dark cerebrospinal fluid (CSF) from an initial 180-degree pulse.)

For cortical processes with mild blood-barrier breakdown or for leptomeningeal disease, enhanced FLAIR images are more sensitive than unenhanced FLAIR or enhanced T1-weighted images. This is probably due to leakage of a small amount of gadolinium into the sulci, which shortens the T1 of the CSF so that it is no longer nulled by the 180-degree pulse on the FLAIR sequence. For this reason, many sites have begun performing FLAIR after contrast is given (rather than before) to increase sensitivity for subtle cortical processes.

Enhancement following the administration of gadolinium extends into the sulci and is therefore leptomeningeal, rather than pachymeningeal. Enhancement of the pachymeninges, i.e., the dura lining the calvarium, the falx, and the tentorium, can be seen in the setting of chronic shunt treatment ("benign meningeal fibrosis"), and following surgery, the enhancement in the latter is localized to the craniotomy site. The differential diagnosis of leptomeningeal enhancement is infectious meningitis and carcinomatous meningitis. Generally, the presence of fever and rapid onset distinguish the infectious from the carcinomatous form.

SUGGESTED READING

Bradley WG, Quencer RM. Hydrocephalus and cerebro-spinal fluid flow. In: Stark DD, Bradley WG, eds. *Magnetic resonance imaging,* 3rd ed. St. Louis: Mosby, 1999:1,483–1,508.

Sze GK. Infection and inflammation. In: Stark DD, Bradley WG, eds. *Magnetic resonance imaging,* 3rd ed. St. Louis: Mosby, 1999:1,361–1,378.

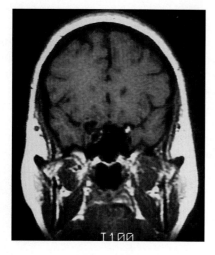

FIG. 85.1A

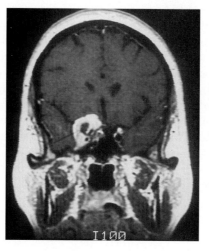

FIG. 85.1B

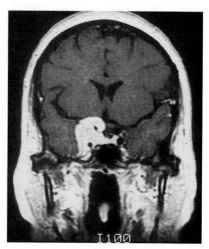

FIG. 85.1C

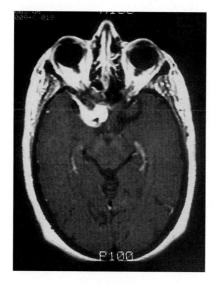

FIG. 85.1D

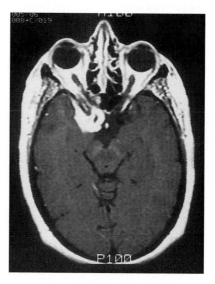

FIG. 85.1E

CLINICAL HISTORY

A 54-year-old woman with decreasing visual acuity in the right eye.

FINDINGS

There is a mass at the right orbital apex, which enhances intensely with gadolinium (Fig. 85.1A–E). The mass narrows the caliber of the cavernous portion of the right internal carotid artery and extends "en plaque" toward the anterior aspect of the right middle cranial fossa. There is also an area of low signal intensity that remains dark following administration of gadolinium (Fig. 85.1A and B). *Submitted by William G. Bradley, M.D., Ph.D., F.A.C.R., Senior Editor, Long Beach Memorial Medical Center, Long Beach, California.*

DIAGNOSIS

Orbital apex meningioma.

DISCUSSION

Parasellar meningiomas are in the differential diagnosis of suprasellar masses. These are characteristically isointense to brain on both T1-weighted (Fig. 85.1A) and T2-weighted images and enhance intensely with gadolinium (Fig. 85.1B–E). Their tendency to narrow the cavernous portion of the internal carotid artery distinguishes them from pituitary macroadenomas, the latter being much softer than the former.

They also have a tendency for thin "en plaque" extension along the dura such that they may only be detectable with gadolinium. Using a combination of coronal (Fig. 85.1D) and axial (Fig. 85.1E) views, involvement of the orbital apex can be confirmed. Meningiomas also tend to develop calcification, which appears as nonenhancing areas of signal void (Fig. 85.1A and B).

SUGGESTED READING

Boyko OB. Adult brain tumors. In: Stark DD, Bradley WG, eds. *Magnetic resonance imaging,* 3rd ed. St. Louis: Mosby, 1999:1,231–1,254.

Zhu M, Maeda M, Lee GJ, et al. Sellar lesions. In: Stark DD, Bradley WG, eds. *Magnetic resonance imaging,* 3rd ed. St. Louis: Mosby, 1999:1,225–1,230.

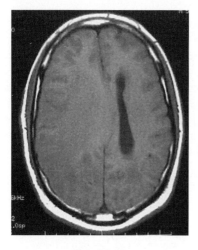

FIG. 86.1A

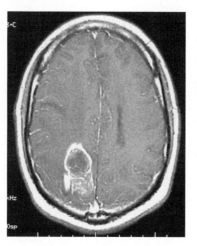

FIG. 86.1B

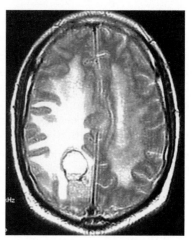

FIG. 86.1C

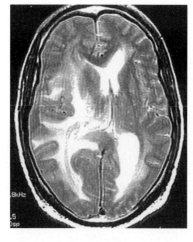

FIG. 86.1D

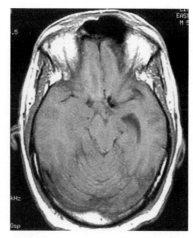

FIG. 86.1E

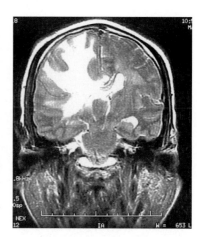

FIG. 86.1F

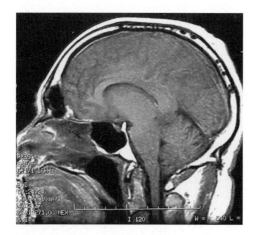

FIG. 86.1G

CLINICAL HISTORY

Elderly patient with headache and left-sided weakness.

FINDINGS

Axial precontrast and postcontrast T1-weighted (Fig. 86.1A and B) and axial T2-weighted images (Fig. 86.1C and D) show a 3-cm heterogeneous, ring-enhancing mass within the right parietal lobe. There is a dependent hypointense fluid level consistent with acute hemorrhage. There is significant perilesional high signal on the T2-weighted acquisition consistent with edema. Note marked shift of the midline structures to the left consistent with subfalcine herniation. There is mass effect upon the right lateral ventricle with dilation and entrapment of the left lateral ventricle. Axial T1-weighted and coronal T2-weighted images (Fig. 86.1E and F) show medial displacement of the right uncus with displacement of the midbrain toward the left, consistent with transtentorial herniation. Sagittal noncontrast T1-weighted acquisition (Fig. 86.1G) shows inferior herniation of the cerebellar tonsils through the foramen magnum.

DIAGNOSIS

Subfalcine, transtentorial, and tonsilar herniation due to hemorrhagic metastasis.

DISCUSSION

The cranial cavity is divided into compartments by bony ridges and dural folds (interhemispheric falx and tentorium). Cerebral herniation is caused by mechanical displacement of brain, cerebrospinal fluid, and blood vessels from one compartment to another. Brain herniation is the sequela of increased intracranial pressure, usually due to an expanding intracranial mass such as traumatic hematoma, edema from infarction, neoplasm, or infectious/inflammatory processes. In addition to the effects of the primary intracranial lesion, the subsequent brain herniation has significant morbidity in and of itself as a result of compression of brain parenchyma, nerves, and/or blood vessels against the bony and dural margins of the cranium. Cerebral herniation often results in severe neurological deficit or death.

There are several types of cerebral herniations, including subfalcine, transtentorial (ascending or descending), transalar, or tonsillar herniation. Subfalcine and descending transtentorial are most frequently encountered.

Subfalcine herniation is the displacement of the cingulate gyrus across the midline under the free inferior edge of the falx cerebri. With larger degrees of midline displacement, there can be compression of the ipsilateral ventricle with contralateral lateral ventricular enlargement due to obstruction of the foramen of Monro. This finding is demonstrated in this case. There may be displacement of the ipsilateral anterior cerebral artery (ACA) across the midline, causing compression of the ACA and its branches against the falx. ACA branch artery occlusion can then result in ischemia and infarction.

There are two types of transtentorial herniation: ascending and descending. The descending type is far more common. In descending transtentorial herniation, the uncus and parahippocampal gyrus of the medial temporal lobe are displaced medially and are seen to protrude over the free tentorial margin. In the early stage, the key imaging finding is effacement of the ipsilateral side of the perimesencephalic and suprasellar cistern. The ipsilateral cerebellopontine angle is widened because of shift of the brainstem away from the herniating temporal lobe. With increasing supratentorial mass effect, there is eventually herniation of both medial temporal lobes, resulting in complete obliteration of the basal cisterns. The tentorial incisura becomes "filled" with both temporal lobes and the lower midbrain. The midbrain becomes compressed and narrowed in its transverse diameter. The medial displacement of the temporal lobes and compression and/or displacement of the brainstem are best seen on coronal MRI (as seen in this case). The anterior choroidal, posterior communicating, and posterior cerebral arteries are also displaced inferomedially in severe descending herniation. Occipital lobe infarction caused by compression of the posterior cerebral artery between the brainstem and the tentorium often occurs with cerebral herniation. Kinking and occlusion of the small perforating vessels can cause infarctions of the basal ganglia and midbrain. Secondary hemorrhages in the midbrain can also occur with transtentorial herniation due to compression of the perforating vessels in the interpeduncular cistern (Duret hemorrhages). "Kernohan notch" is a focus of edema, ischemia, or hemorrhagic necrosis within the cerebral peduncle on the opposite side from the herniating temporal lobe. It is caused by compression of the peduncle against the tentorium as the brainstem is shifted away from the herniating mass. This finding can be associated with ipsilateral hemiparesis.

Ascending transtentorial herniation is the upward herniation of the vermis and cerebellar hemispheres through the tentorial incisura. It is associated with infratentorial traumatic injury or significant perilesional mass effect and is therefore much less common than the descending type. On imaging, the superior cerebellar cistern and fourth ventricles are compressed. The quadrigeminal cistern and midbrain may be compressed and/or displaced. Obstructive hydrocephalus may occur due to aqueductal obstruction.

Tonsillar herniation is the inferior displacement of the cerebellar tonsils through the foramen magnum and is best seen on sagittal MRI. It occurs in two thirds of patients with ascending transtentorial herniation and in half of cases of descending transtentorial herniation.

Descending transalar herniation is an uncommon form of cerebral herniation in which the frontal lobe is displaced posteriorly over the greater sphenoid ridge, causing backward displacement of the sylvian fissure, the middle cerebral artery, and the temporal lobe. In ascending transalar herniation, the temporal lobe, sylvian fissure, and middle cerebral artery are pushed up and over the sphenoid ridge.

SUGGESTED READING

Laine FJ, Shedden AI, Dunn MM, et al. Acquired intracranial herniations: MR imaging findings. *AJR* 1995; 165(4):967–973.

Osborn AG. Secondary effects of intracranial trauma. *Neurosurg Clin North Am* 1991;1:461–474.

Reich JB, Sierra J, Camp W, et al. Magnetic resonance imaging measurements and clinical changes accompanying transtentorial and foramen magnum brain herniation. *Ann Neurol* 1993;33(2):159–170.

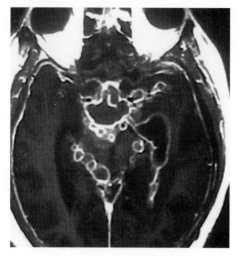 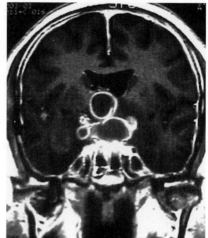

FIG. 87.1A   **FIG. 87.1B**

CLINICAL HISTORY

A 45-year-old East Indian man with lethargy and confusion.

FINDINGS

Axial and coronal postcontrast T1-weighted images (Fig. 87.1A and B) demonstrate smooth abnormal thickening of the meninges over the cerebral convexities and temporal lobes. There are multiloculated peripherally enhancing masses in the suprasellar and basal cisterns.

DIAGNOSIS

Tuberculosis (TB) meningitis.

DISCUSSION

In recent years, the incidence of TB is rising, particularly among immigrants, the homeless, intravenous drug abusers, human immunodeficiency virus–infected, and institutionalized patients. *Mycobacterium tuberculosis* is the responsible organism in the vast majority of cases. *Mycobacterium avium-intracellulare complex* rarely involves the central nervous system (CNS). Most adult CNS TB is a postprimary infection, whereas in children, it is usually part of a primary infection. CNS TB occurs in 2% to 5% of all patients with TB, and in 10% of those with acquired immunodeficiency syndrome–related TB infection. In post–primary infection, it is postulated that the organism is transported to the meninges and/or brain parenchyma hematogenously from a primary pulmonary TB infection. Coexistent pulmonary TB is seen in 25% to 83% of cases of CNS TB.

Various manifestations of CNS TB include TB meningitis, parenchymal abscess, focal cerebritis, and tuberculoma.

TB meningitis (as seen in this case) is typically a chronic, indolent meningeal process, although an active form does occur. The patient typically presents with fever, headache, mental status change, and meningeal signs. The organism forms a thick, gelatinous exudate that predominantly involves the basal cisterns, although there can be more diffuse involvement. Approximately 17.5% of all CNS TB infection is isolated to the meninges. Vascular thromboses and/or occlusion often occur (28% to 41% of cases) at the base of the brain due to the direct effect of the tuberculous exudate and/or a reactive endarteritis obliterans. The middle cerebral artery and its branches (especially the medial lenticulostriate vessels supplying the basal ganglia) are most often affected. This accounts for the characteristic bilateral basal ganglia infarcts frequently seen in the setting of TB meningitis.

Active TB meningitis is most conspicuous on postcontrast T1-weighted images, which demonstrate diffuse meningeal enhancement. Chronic meningitis shows characteristic thickened, enhancing basilar meninges, seen on both contrast-enhanced CT and T1-weighted images. Coarse "popcorn-like" calcifications can be seen, particularly around the basal cisterns on CT. These calcified meningeal nodules are hypointense on all MRI pulse sequences and often demonstrate peripheral enhancement. Meningeal enhancement can persist for years after the initial diagnosis and treatment of TB meningitis.

Bilateral infarctions occur in 70% of cases. Most infarcts are seen in the medial lenticulostriate and thalamoperforator artery territories and are detected earlier on MRI. Some involve the cerebral cortex. Hydrocephalus is a common associated finding.

TB meningitis can also present as a focal ("en plaque") dural-based enhancing mass. These lesions are often slightly hyperdense on CT, isointense on T1-weighted images, and isointense to hypointense on T2-weighted images.

The overall mortality rate in TB meningitis is 25% to 30% with significant morbidity in long-term survivors.

Differential diagnosis for chronic basilar meningitis, as seen in this case, includes *Coccidioides immitis* and *Cryptococcus neoformans*. Sarcoidosis and carcinomatous meningitis could have a similar appearance. Focal "en plaque" disease can mimic meningioma, dural lymphoma, or sarcoidosis.

SUGGESTED READING

Chang KH, Han MH, Roh JK, et al. Gd-DTPA enhanced MR imaging in intracranial tuberculosis. *Neuroradiology* 1991;238:340–344.

Goyal M, Sharma A, Mishra NK, et al. Imaging appearance of pachymeningeal tuberculosis. *AJR* 1997; 169(5):1,421–1,424.

Hansman Whiteman ML, Bowen BC, Donovan Post MJ, et al. Intracranial infection. In: Atlas SW, ed. *Magnetic resonance imaging of the brain and spine,* 2nd ed. Philadelphia: Lippincott–Raven Publishers, 1996:738–742.

Hsieh FY, Chia LG, Shen WC. Locations of cerebral infarctions in tuberculous meningitis. *Neuroradiology* 1992;34:197–199.

Jinkins JR. Computed tomography of intracranial tuberculosis. *Neuroradiology* 1991;33:126–135.

Kloumehr F, Dadsetan MR, Rooholamini SA, et al. Central nervous system tuberculosis: MRI. *Neuroradiology* 1994;36(2):93–96.

Sheller JR, DesPrez RM. CNS tuberculosis. *Neurol Clin* 1986;4:143–158.

Tayfun C, Ucoz T, Tasar M, et al. Diagnostic value of MRI in tuberculous meningitis. *Eur Radiol* 1996;6(3):380–386.

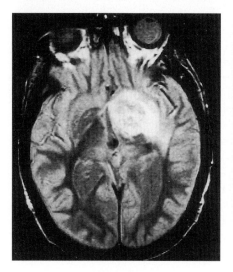

FIG. 88.1A

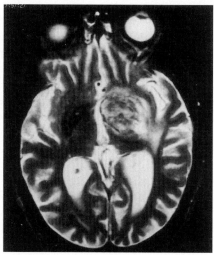

FIG. 88.1B

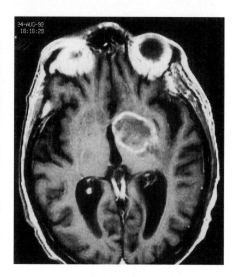

FIG. 88.1C

CLINICAL HISTORY

A 37-year-old man with acquired immunodeficiency syndrome (AIDS) presents with decreasing level of consciousness.

FINDINGS

Proton density (Fig. 88.1A) and T2-weighted (Fig. 88.1B) images through the basal ganglia demonstrate a hypointense lesion with surrounding hyperintense vasogenic edema. Following administration of gadolinium, a T1-weighted image (Fig. 88.1C) demonstrates an enhancing border. *Submitted by William G. Bradley, M.D., Ph.D., F.A.C.R., Senior Editor, Long Beach Memorial Medical Center, Long Beach, California.*

DIAGNOSIS

Lymphoma.

DISCUSSION

Primary central nervous system (CNS) lymphoma is frequently central in location, particularly in AIDS patients. On T2-weighted images, lymphoma is typically hypointense, reflecting the high nuclear-cytoplasmic ratio. This feature may be useful in distinguishing it from a glioblastoma multiforme, which is generally hyperintense centrally on a T2-weighted image. Necrotic lymphoma may be impossible to distinguish from glioblastoma multiforme or from abscess, particularly in AIDS patients. In such cases, spectroscopy may be useful, demonstrating elevated choline level in lymphoma or glioblastoma multiforme glomerular basement basement membrane (GBM) and absent choline in toxoplasmosis or other abscess.

SUGGESTED READING

Boyko OB. Adult brain tumors. In: Stark DD, Bradley WG, eds. *Magnetic resonance imaging,* 3rd ed. St. Louis: Mosby, 1999:1231–1254.

Danielsen ER, Ross BD. Neurospectroscopy. In: Stark DD, Bradley WG, eds. *Magnetic resonance imaging,* 3rd ed. St. Louis: Mosby, 1999:1,595–1,636.

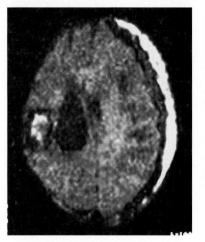

FIG. 89.1A

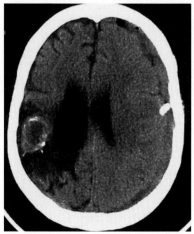

FIG. 89.1B

CLINICAL HISTORY

A 56-year-old woman with history of head trauma.

FINDINGS

Axial diffusion-weighted MRI acquisition (Fig. 89.1A) demonstrates an abnormal extraaxial collection of high signal over the left cerebral convexity consistent with subdural hematoma. There is perifocal mass effect with effacement of underlying cortical sulci and shift of midline structures toward the right. Additionally, there is a rounded focus of high signal with surrounding low signal within the right posterior frontal/parietal lobe. Axial noncontrast CT scan

(Fig. 89.1B) confirms the subdural hematoma. The focus of signal abnormality seen on the diffusion-weighted image shows foci of dystrophic calcification in an area of encephalomalacia. There is diffuse low density involving the cortex and subcortical white matter of the right posterior frontal and parietal lobes suggestive of old cortical infarct in the right middle cerebral artery distribution.

DIAGNOSIS

Subdural hematoma with "misleading focus" of high signal on the diffusion-weighted image.

DISCUSSION

In the vast majority of cases, calcium is seen as a focus of signal void on MRI images, due to its lack of signal-yielding hydrogen nuclei. Occasionally, cases of floccular calcification within the brain parenchyma can lead to T1 shortening of relaxation for adjacent hydrogen nuclei on the basis of surface-layer absorption effects similar to those seen with highly proteinaceous fluid (such as edema associated with acutely demyelinating lesions or in inspissated mucus). This T1 shortening effect can be observed not only on T1-weighted images, but also on T2-weighted and fluid-attenuated inversion-recovery images. Differentiation from hemorrhage in the methemoglobin stage may be impossible in such cases (as with CT when floccular calcium can mimic the high density of blood).

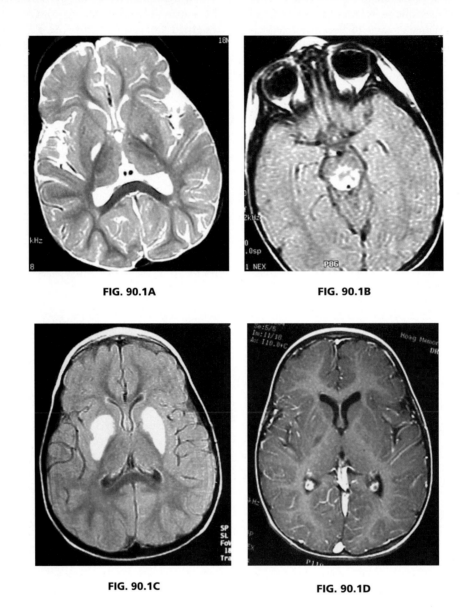

FIG. 90.1A　　　　**FIG. 90.1B**

FIG. 90.1C　　　　**FIG. 90.1D**

CLINICAL HISTORY

A 2-year-old girl with history of ataxia, hypotonia, and nystagmus.

FINDINGS

Initial MRI of the brain demonstrates marked abnormal high signal within the globus pallidus bilaterally extending down into the dorsal aspect of the brainstem at the level of the midbrain and pons with involvement of the periaqueductal gray matter on the axial T2-weighted (Fig. 90.1A) and fluid-attenuated inversion-recovery (FLAIR) acquisitions (Fig. 90.1B). Two-year follow-up study axial FLAIR (Fig. 90.1C) demonstrates dramatic increase in the extent of signal abnormality now involving the putamen and globus pallidus bilaterally. Postcontrast T1-weighted images (Fig. 90.1D) demonstrate no abnormal intracranial enhancement.

DIAGNOSIS

Leigh disease.

DISCUSSION

Leigh disease is a member of the group of inherited diseases known as the "mitochondrial encephalopathies." Also included in this group are MELAS (mitochondrial myopathy, encephalopathy, lactic acidosis, and strokelike episodes), MERRF (myoclonic epilepsy with ragged red fiber myopathy), and Kearns-Sayre syndrome, among others. These entities are characterized by mitochondrial defects that result in impaired adenosine triphosphate production in affected cells. Single or multiple organs can be affected, with the striated muscle and brain most commonly involved.

Leigh disease (subacute necrotizing encephalopathy) represents end-stage mitochondrial dysfunction. It is a rare, autosomal recessive disorder. Affected infants and children usually present with hypotonia and psychomotor deterioration. Other reported symptoms include ataxia, dystonia, seizures, and visual loss. The infantile form of disease is the most common and usually presents before the age of 2. There are also juvenile and adult forms of Leigh disease, which manifest in early childhood and in the fifth and sixth decades, respectively. Death usually ensues within a few years of symptom onset, usually due to respiratory arrest.

Pathologically, Leigh disease is characterized by microcystic cavitation, capillary proliferation, neuronal loss and demyelination, with primary involvement of the midbrain, basal ganglia, and cerebellar dentate nuclei. The periaqueductal, subependymal, and tegmental gray matter are commonly involved. Occasionally, the cerebral white matter is affected.

On nonenhanced CT, the disease presents as low-density areas in the putamina and caudate nuclei. The lesions do not typically enhance. The findings on T2-weighted MRI scans are striking with intense, symmetric hyperintense foci, usually involving the basal ganglia, periaqueductal gray matter, cerebral peduncles, and thalami. Signal abnormality within the putamina is the most consistently reported finding in Leigh disease, most often affecting the anterior aspect. The caudate nuclei, globus pallidi, and thalami are frequently affected, but not in the absence of putamen disease. The cortical gray matter, the superior cerebellar peduncles, the cerebral white matter, and the posterior columns of the spinal cord are less commonly involved. Significant demyelination may be present but is very uncommon. Enlarged, edematous basal ganglia and thalami have been reported in the acute/subacute stage of disease. Hyperintense foci on T1-weighted images can be seen in the acute stage due to acute necrosis and hemorrhage. Noteworthy are the characteristic magnetic resonance spectroscopy findings of decreased neutron activation analysis (NAA) levels and elevated lactate levels in patients with Leigh disease. This is in contrast to the lack of a lactate peak in patients with nonmitochondrial disorders affecting the basal ganglia, such as Wilson disease and chronic infarction. Wernicke encephalopathy can have a similar pathologic and imaging appearance. The lack of mammillary body involvement in Leigh disease is an important differential diagnostic feature.

SUGGESTED READING

Barkovich AJ. *Pediatric neuroimaging,* 2nd ed. Philadelphia: Lippincott–Raven Publishers, 1996:94–96.

Lexa FJ, Trojanowski JQ, Braffman BH, et al. The aging brain and neurodegenerative diseases. In: Atlas SW, ed. *Magnetic resonance imaging of the brain and spine,* 2nd ed. Philadelphia: Lippincott–Raven Publishers, 1996:849–850.

Medina L, Chi T, DeVivo D, et al. MR findings in patients with subacute necrotizing encephalopathy (Leigh disease): correlation with biochemical defect. *AJNR* 1990;11:379–384.

Valanne L, Ketonen L, Majender A, et al. Neuroradiology findings in children with mitochondrial disease. *AJNR* 1998;19:369–377.

Zimmerman RA, Wang ZJ. The value of proton MR spectroscopy in pediatric metabolic brain disease. *AJNR* 1997;18:1872–1879.

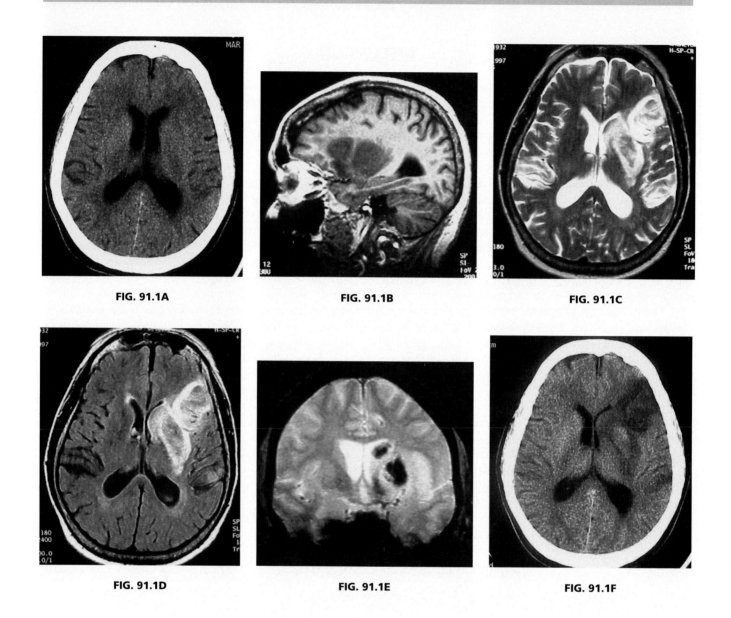

FIG. 91.1A **FIG. 91.1B** **FIG. 91.1C**

FIG. 91.1D **FIG. 91.1E** **FIG. 91.1F**

CLINICAL HISTORY

A 64-year-old woman with sudden right hemiparesis.

FINDINGS

Axial noncontrast CT images on the day of presentation (Fig. 91.1A) demonstrated no significant abnormality. Within the following 24 hours, an MRI was performed. Noncontrast T1-weighted image (Fig. 91.1B) demonstrates a large region of hypointense signal involving the left frontal operculum and basal ganglia. Axial T2-weighted and fluid-attenuated inversion-recovery images (Fig. 91.1C and D) show a large region of high signal in a similar distribution consistent with acute infarct. Coronal gradient echo acquisition (Fig. 91.1E) shows central low signal magnetic susceptibility effect due to hemorrhagic conversion.

DIAGNOSIS

Acute infarct with hemorrhagic transformation.

DISCUSSION

Hemorrhagic conversion of acute ischemic infarction can be seen in approximately 25% to 30% of all acute middle cerebral artery infarcts within the first 3 days. This is due to reperfusion of the ischemic brain region, and its loss of blood–brain barrier integrity. Reintroduction of systemic blood pressure into this damaged vascular bed, which cannot autoregulate (unlike normal brain vasculature) in the face of sudden blood pressure spikes, leads to this hemorrhagic conversion. Such hemorrhage often causes clinical deterioration. Because of this, systemic anticoagulation is generally withheld in large infarcts of the middle cerebral artery.

Gradient recalled sequences are particularly sensitive to brain parenchymal hemorrhage and match the sensitivity of CT for detection of blood products in the early stages; this sensitivity is due to the inhomogeneity of magnetic fields caused by the deoxyhemoglobin molecule, which is strongly paramagnetic. Dephasing of spins in the face of magnetic field inhomogeneity leads to the signal loss observable on gradient recalled sequences.

Many infarcts will show small zones of hemorrhagic conversion in the 10-to-20-day time frame. These are usually of no clinical consequence and do not contraindicate use of anticoagulants.

On the following day, a repeated noncontrast CT image was acquired (Fig. 91.1F), which demonstrated acute infarct within the left frontal operculum and hemorrhagic conversion.

SUGGESTED READING

Hasso AN, Stringer WA, Brown KD. Cerebral ischemia and infarction. *Neuroimaging Clin North Am* 1994;4(4): 733–752.

Larrue V, von Kummer R, del Zoppo G, et al. Hemorrhagic transformation in acute ischemic stroke. *Stroke* 1997;28:957–960.

Motto C, Ciccone A, Aritzu E, et al. Hemorrhage after an acute ischemic stroke. *Stroke* 1999;30:761–764.

Weingarten K, Filippi C, Zimmerman RD, et al. Detection of hemorrhage in acute cerebral infarction: evaluation with spin-echo and gradient-echo MRI. *Clin Imaging* 1994;18(1):43–55.

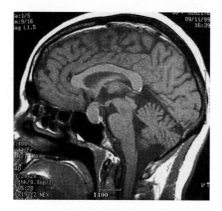

FIG. 92.1A

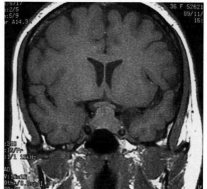

FIG. 92.1B

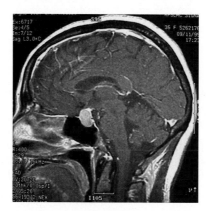

FIG. 92.1C

CLINICAL HISTORY

A 36-year-old postpartum woman with recent decreased visual acuity.

FINDINGS

Sagittal and coronal T1-weighted images (Fig. 92.1A and B) demonstrate enlargement of the pituitary gland with suprasellar extension. The mass is homogeneous and intermediate in signal. Following intravenous contrast (Fig. 92.1C), there is mild homogeneous enhancement. There is mild mass effect upon the undersurface of the optic chiasm. There is no extension into the cavernous sinus. *Figures 92.1A–C courtesy of Cornel Overbeeker, M.D., Rush-Presbyterian-St. Luke's Medical Center; Chicago, Illinois.*

DIAGNOSIS

Lymphocytic hypophysitis (LH).

DISCUSSION

LH is a rare, noninfectious, inflammatory disorder of the pituitary gland. The disorder characteristically involves the anterior pituitary gland and is thought to be immune mediated. Many affected patients have concurrent autoimmune endocrinologic disorders such as Hashimoto thyroiditis or Grave disease. Histopathologically, there is lymphocytic infiltration of the adenohypophysis with occasional plasma cells. This chronic inflammatory process eventually leads to fibrosis and pituitary gland atrophy.

LH occurs primarily in young women, particularly during pregnancy or the postpartum period. LH has, however, been rarely reported in men and in postmenopausal women. Patients often present with headache, visual loss, amenorrhea, and/or inability to lactate. Pituitary hormone production (i.e., prolactin) is usually diminished; however, elevated levels have been reported.

Typical imaging features of LH include an enlarged homogeneously enhancing intrasellar mass with suprasellar extension, as seen in this case. Differentiation from pituitary macroadenoma is impossible radiographically. There are usually no focal intrinsic lesions; the internal architecture of the enlarged gland is homogeneous. Delayed enhancement of the pituitary mass has been reported in LH as compared with a normal gland. Heterogeneous enhancement of the gland and cavernous sinus involvement has been reported. Given normal physiologic enlargement of the pituitary gland during pregnancy, the diagnosis can be difficult. The normal gland in late pregnancy can reach 12 to 13 mm in size. It typically has a spherical contour with convex superior margin. One study suggests that intense enhancement of the gland and adjacent dural enhancement should suggest the diagnosis of LH.

In classic LH, disease is confined to the adenohypophysis. Cases of posterior pituitary gland and stalk involvement have been described in patients with diabetes insipidus. This relatively newly described entity is referred to as "lymphocytic infundibuloneurohypophysitis."

LH patients often improve with steroid treatment. There can be spontaneous resolution.

SUGGESTED READING

Kojima H, Nojima T, Nagashama K, et al. Diabetes insipidus caused by lymphocytic infundibuloneurohypophysitis. *Arch Pathol Lab Med* 1989;113:1,399–1,401.

Nussbaume CE, Okawara S, Jacobs LS. Lymphocytic hypophysitis with involvement of the cavernous sinus and hypothalamus. *Neurosurgery* 1991;28:440–444.

Quencer RM. Lymphocytic adenohypophysitis: autoimmune disorder of the pituitary gland. *AJNR* 1980;1:343–345.

Saiwai S, Inoue Y, Ishihara T. Lymphocytic adenohypophysitis: skull radiographs and MRI. *Neuroradiology* 1998; 40:114–120.

Sato N, Sze G, Endo K. Hypophysitis: endrocrinologic and dynamic MR findings. *AJNR* 1998;19:439–444.

Supler ML, Mickls JP. Lymphocytic hypophysitis: report of a case in a man with cavernous sinus involvement. *Surg Neurol* 1992;37:472–476.

Thodou E, Asa SL, Kontogeorgos G, et al. Clinical case seminar: lymphocytic hypophysitis: clinicopathological findings. *J Clin Endocrinol Metab* 1995;80(8):2,302–2,311.

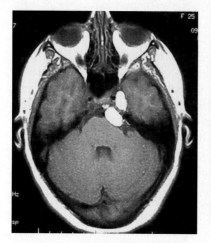

FIG. 93.1A

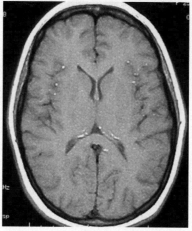

FIG. 93.1B

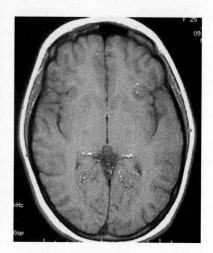

FIG. 93.1C

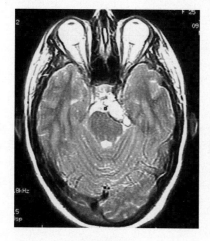

FIG. 93.1D

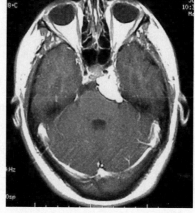

FIG. 93.1E

CLINICAL HISTORY

A 25-year-old woman with left-sided facial pain.

FINDINGS

Axial noncontrast T1-weighted image (Fig. 93.1A) demonstrates a large lobulated hyperintense mass within the left cerebellar pontine angle along the cisternal portion of the left fifth cranial nerve. There is extension of tumor into the region of Meckel cave. More superiorly (Fig. 93.1B and C), there are tiny foci of high signal on this T1-weighted image within the sulci of the sylvian fissures bilaterally, as well as along the ependymal surface of the lateral ventricles. Axial fast spin echo T2-weighted image (Fig. 93.1D) shows the mass is hyperintense but less intense than on the T1-weighted acquisition. Note the chemical shift artifact in the frequency (anteroposterior) direction. Following intravenous contrast (Fig. 93.1E), there is no significant enhancement.

DIAGNOSIS

Ruptured dermoid tumor.

DISCUSSION

Dermoid tumors are congenital lesions that result from the inclusion of epithelium at the time of neural tube closure in embryogenesis. They are rare, slow-growing, cystic tumors that are typically located in the midline.

Dermoid cysts are lobulated cystic masses that contain thick, viscous oily fluid composed of lipid metabolites and liquid cholesterol (derived from decomposed epithelial cells). The outer wall is composed of dense fibrous tissue; the interior is lined by squamous epithelium, hair, and dermal appendages (hair follicles, sebaceous and sweat glands). Calcification is common, either dystrophic or related to dental enamel (an ectodermal derivative). The common misconception is that dermoids contain both ectodermal and mesodermal elements while epidermoid tumors contain only ectodermal elements. The fact is that both dermoid and epidermoid tumors are ectodermal inclusion cysts. Although hair, sebaceous, and sweat glands lie within mesodermal connective tissue, these dermal appendages actually arise from embryonic ectoderm.

Most commonly found in the lumbosacral canal, intracranial dermoids can occur in the posterior fossa within the cerebellopontine angle (as seen in this case), the midline vermis, or fourth ventricle. Dermoids can also occur in the parasellar and frontobasal regions. Symptoms usually result from compression of adjacent neural structures, with seizures and headache being the common presenting complaints. Occasionally, the cyst ruptures, causing a diffuse chemical meningitis.

Dermoid tumors appear as well-defined hypodense masses on CT with Hounsfield unit measurements of −0 to −40. Calcification is common. Hyperdense lesions have been reported but are rare.

On MRI, dermoid tumors demonstrate high signal on T1-weighted images, reflecting their fat content. They have variable signal on T2-weighted images. Enhancement is uncommon. If the cyst has ruptured (as seen in this case), multiple tiny foci of high-signal fat droplets on T1-weighted images are seen scattered throughout the subarachnoid space. Classic fat–cerebrospinal fluid levels may be seen within the nondependent portion of the lateral ventricles.

The differential diagnosis is primarily intracranial lipoma. The presence of material other than fat within the lesion distinguishes a dermoid tumor from intracranial lipoma. Dermoids without fat or calcification can mimic an epidermoid or arachnoid cyst.

SUGGESTED READING

Drolshagen LF, Standefer M. Dense dermoid cyst of the posterior fossa. *AJNR* 1991;12:317.

Lunardi P, Missori P. Supratentorial dermoid cysts. *J Neurosurg* 1991;75:262–266.

Osborn AG. Miscellaneous tumors, cysts, and metastases. In: *Diagnostic neuroradiology,* 1st ed. St.Louis: Mosby, 1994:635–636.

Smith AS. Myth of the mesoderm: ectodermal origin of dermoids. *AJNR* 1989;10:449.

Wilms G, Casselman J, Demaerel P, et al. CT and MRI of ruptured intracranial dermoids. *Neuroradiology* 1991; 33(2):149–151.

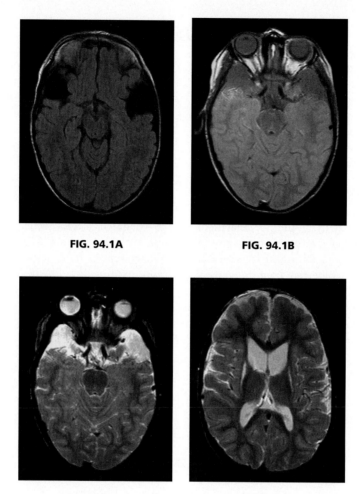

FIG. 94.1A

FIG. 94.1B

FIG. 94.1C

FIG. 94.1D

CLINICAL HISTORY

A 4-year-old boy with mental retardation and worsening movement disorder.

FINDINGS

Bilateral middle cranial fossa extraaxial fluid collections are present (Fig. 94.1A–C). There is dilation of the sylvian fissures bilaterally. There is increased signal intensity in both basal ganglia on T2-weighted fluid-attenuated inversion-recovery images (Fig. 94.1D). *Submitted by George Rappard, M.D., University of California, Irvine, Orange, California; and William G. Bradley, M.D., Ph.D., F.A.C.R., Senior Editor, Long Beach Memorial Medical Center, Long Beach, California.*

DIAGNOSIS

Glutaric aciduria.

DISCUSSION

Glutaric aciduria type I (GA-I) is an uncommon autosomal recessive metabolic disorder due to a deficiency of glutaryl-CoA dehydrogenase. This enzyme is responsible for the metabolism of L-lysine, hydroxy-L-lysine, and L-tryptophan. Patients with GA-I present with intermittent or chronic metabolic acidemia, movement disorder, and mental retardation. The movement disorder is characterized as progressive choreoathetosis, hyperkinesia, and spasticity. Some individuals, however, are asymptomatic. Laboratory evaluation reveals large amounts of glutaric acid and β-hydroxyglutarate in the urine, as well as generalized aminoaciduria.

The mechanism for neurological deterioration in GA-I is theorized to be due to inhibition of neuronal glutamate decarboxylase. β-hydroxyglutarate and glutaric acid are both potent inhibitors of this enzyme. Biochemical analysis has revealed elevated levels of glutaric acid in the frontal cortex and basal ganglia.

MRI of patients with GA-I reveals bat-wing dilation of the sylvian fissures. Some authors have considered this to be secondary to frontotemporal atrophy while others feel this is due to frontotemporal hypoplasia. Imaging of the temporal lobes may reveal that they are normal or may reveal coronally oriented white matter on axial images, normal cortical thickness, and loss of parenchyma. These findings are consistent with hypoplasia or hypogenesis of the temporal lobes. There is improvement in the appearance of the temporal lobes after therapy with oral carnitine. In addition, there is dilation of the cerebrospinal fluid space surrounding the temporal lobes. These have the radiologic appearance of middle cranial fossa arachnoid cysts. These arachnoid cysts may be associated with temporal lobe hypogenesis. One author postulates that they may be secondary to the occurrence of a severe and rapid frontotemporal atrophy. Bilateral, symmetric demyelination is a consistent finding. The basal ganglia may be small, atrophic, or increased in signal intensity on T2-weighted images. Despite prominent choreoathetosis, radiologic involvement of the basal ganglia may be minimal. Diffuse cortical atrophy, bilateral subdural hygromas, and hematomas and prominent mesencephalic cisterns have been reported.

SUGGESTED READING

Altman NR, Rovira MJ, Bauer M. Glutaric aciduria type I: MR findings in two cases. *AJNR* 1991;12:966–968.

Goodman SI, Norenberg MD, Shikes RH, et al. Glutaric aciduria: biochemical and morphologic considerations. *J Pediatr* 1977;90:746–750.

Hald JK, Nakstad PH, Skjeldal OH, et al. Bilateral arachnoid cysts of the temporal fossa in four children with glutaric aciduria type I. *AJNR* 1991;12:407–409.

Mandel H, Braun J, El-Peleg O, et al. Glutaric aciduria type I. Brain CT features and diagnostic pitfalls. *Neuroradiology* 1991;33:75–78.

Naidu S, Moser HW. Value of neuroimaging in metabolic diseases affecting the CNS. *AJNR* 1991;12:413–416.

Osborn A. *Diagnostic neuroradiology.* St. Louis: Mosby, 1994.

Stokke O, Goodman SI, Moe PG. Inhibition of brain glutamate decarboxylase by glutarate, glutaconate, and beta-hydroxyglutarate: explanation of the symptoms in glutaric aciduria? *Clin Chim Acta* 1976;66:411–415.

Wu JY, Roberts E. Properties of brain I-glutamate decarboxylase: inhibition studies. *J Neurochem* 1974;23:759–767.

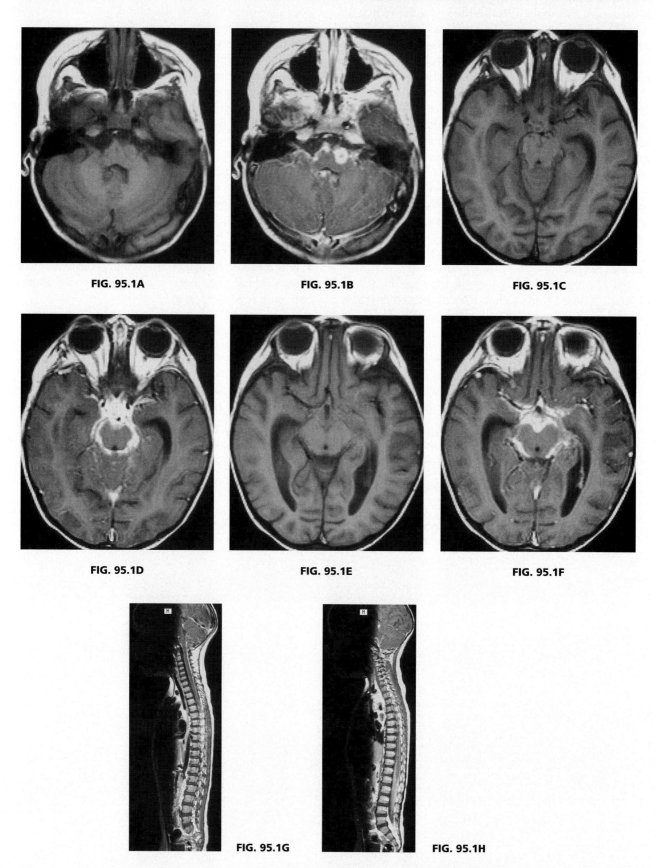

FIG. 95.1A

FIG. 95.1B

FIG. 95.1C

FIG. 95.1D

FIG. 95.1E

FIG. 95.1F

FIG. 95.1G

FIG. 95.1H

CLINICAL HISTORY

A 2-year-old Indian boy with lethargy progressing to coma.

FINDINGS

There is dense meningeal enhancement in the basal cisterns with essentially no involvement of the subarachnoid space over the basal convexities (Fig. 95.1A–F). The enhancement also involves the spinal subarachnoid space (Fig. 95.1G and H). *Submitted by William G. Bradley, M.D., Ph.D., F.A.C.R., Senior Editor, Long Beach Memorial Medical Center, Long Beach, California.*

DIAGNOSIS

Tuberculosis (TB) meningitis.

DISCUSSION

The differential diagnosis of meningeal enhancement can be first divided on the basis of whether enhancement involves the pachymeninges (dura) or the leptomeninges (pia and arachnoid). Enhancement of the former involves the dura over the convexities as well as the falx and the tentorium. This does not extend into the sulci or the subarachnoid cisterns and can be seen in the setting of long-term shunt therapy (benign meningeal fibrosis). Leptomeningeal enhancement, on the other hand, extends into the sulci.

The differential diagnosis of leptomeningeal enhancement is leptomeningeal carcinomatosis and meningitis. While these sarcoid conditions are generally distinguishable on the basis of their clinical presentation, they can have a similar appearance, particularly for severe viral or bacterial meningitis. Fungal meningitis and TB meningitis, on the other hand, tend to involve the basal cisterns, which often provides a key to the diagnosis (Fig. 95.1B, D, and F). Because of the thick purulent exudate in the basal cisterns, cerebrospinal fluid flow beyond the outlet foramina of the fourth ventricle (Luschka and Magendie) is obstructed, leading to communicating hydrocephalus.

SUGGESTED READING

Sze GB. Infection and inflammation. In: Stark DD, Bradley WG, eds. *Magnetic resonance imaging*, 3rd ed. St. Louis: Mosby, 1999:1,361–1,378.

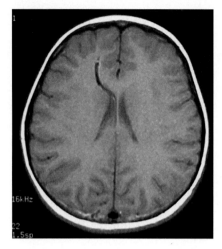

FIG. 96.1A

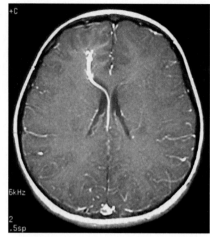

FIG. 96.1B

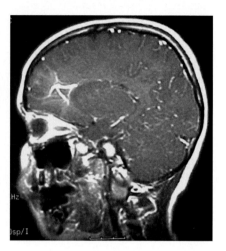

FIG. 96.1C

CLINICAL HISTORY

Headache.

FINDINGS

Axial T1-weighted acquisition demonstrates a linear region of low signal within the right frontal lobe extending to the frontal horn of the right lateral ventricle (Fig. 96.1A). Axial and sagittal post-contrast images (Fig. 96.1B and C) demonstrate several tiny linear enhancing structures within the right frontal lobe, which drain into the large enhancing medullary vein in a "caput medusae" pattern. The medullary vein courses along the ependymal surface of the right lateral ventricle toward the internal cerebral veins. *Figures 96.1A–C courtesy of Sri Kannan, M.D., Rush-Presbyterian-St. Luke's Medical Center, Chicago, Illinois.*

DIAGNOSIS

Venous angioma.

DISCUSSION

Venous angioma may be missed on MRI images without the use of intravenous contrast but can be a source of unnecessary concern when found on postcontrast images and not identified as such. The classic appearance of a branching serpentine structure, which typically drains into a single layer vein, is the major clue. Occasionally, on conventional T2-weighted images, phase-displacement artifact can demonstrate this branching pattern without the use of intravenous contrast. Venous angioma is a clinically inconsequential condition in the vast majority of cases; occasionally, it can be associated with capillary angioma and/or foci of hemorrhage. Angiography confirms the presence of venous angioma but is rarely necessary—the venous phase of the angiogram showing the abnormal venous structure with the multiple draining veins coalescing centrally (Medusa head appearance).

SUGGESTED READING

Field LR, Russell EJ. Spontaneous hemorrhage from a cerebral venous malformation related to thrombosis of the central draining vein: demonstration with angiography and serial MR. *AJNR* 1995;16:1,885–1,888.

Goulao A, Alvarez H, Monaco RG, et al. Venous anomalies and abnormalities of the posterior fossa. *Neuroradiology* 1990;31:476–482.

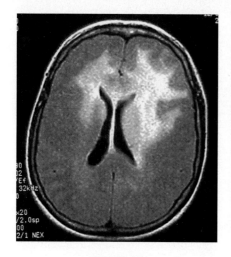

FIG. 97.1A

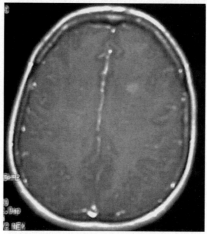

FIG. 97.1B

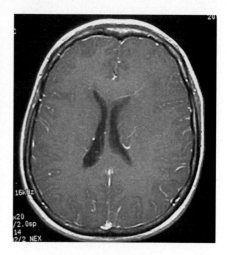

FIG. 97.1C

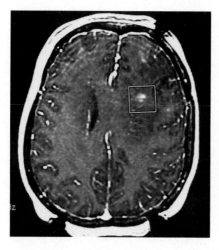

FIG. 97.1D

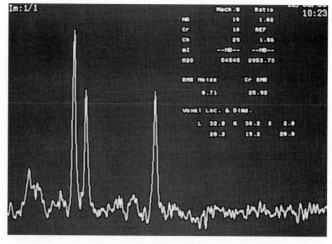

FIG. 97.1E

CLINICAL HISTORY

A 44-year-old woman with headaches and personality change.

FINDINGS

Axial fluid-attenuated inversion-recovery acquisition (Fig. 97.1A) demonstrates confluent abnormal high signal within the deep periventricular and subcortical white matter of both frontal lobes with extension across the corpus callosum. There is thickening and increased signal within the septum pellucidum. Following intravenous contrast, the T1-weighted image (Fig. 97.1B and C) shows a subtle, tiny focus of enhancement within the left centrum semiovale. The bulk of the lesion does not enhance. Magnetic resonance spectroscopy (Fig. 97.1D and E) demonstrates elevated creatine and choline peaks with diminution of N-acetylcholine.

DIAGNOSIS

Gliomatosis cerebri.

DISCUSSION

The diffuse nature of the lesion with relatively little mass effect, the fact that there is extension across the corpus callosum (unusual in any other lesions except for primary white matter disease or radiation effect), and the relatively insidious onset of the clinical findings are clues to the diagnosis. Gliomatosis cerebri can be extremely diffuse throughout the brain. Dedifferentiation into more malignant astrocytomas eventually occurs but may take years to develop. Magnetic resonance spectroscopy is a very helpful tool in detecting the loss of normal N-acetylaspartate with these conditions, as well as elevation of choline caused by the relatively rapid cell-membrane turnover and breakdown associated with astrocytoma. Although not always specific for astrocytoma, this characteristic spectroscopic pattern is strongly confirmatory of astrocytoma.

SUGGESTED READING

del Carpio-O'Donovan R, Korah I, Salazar A, et al. Gliomatosis cerebri. *Radiology* 1996;198:831–835.

Felsberg GJ, Silver SA, Brown MT, et al. Radiologic-pathologic correlation gliomatosis cerebri. *AJNR* 1994; 15:1,745–1,753.

Spagnoli MV, Grossman RI, Packer RJ, et al. Magnetic resonance imaging determination of gliomatosis cerebri. *Neuroradiology* 1987;29:15–18.

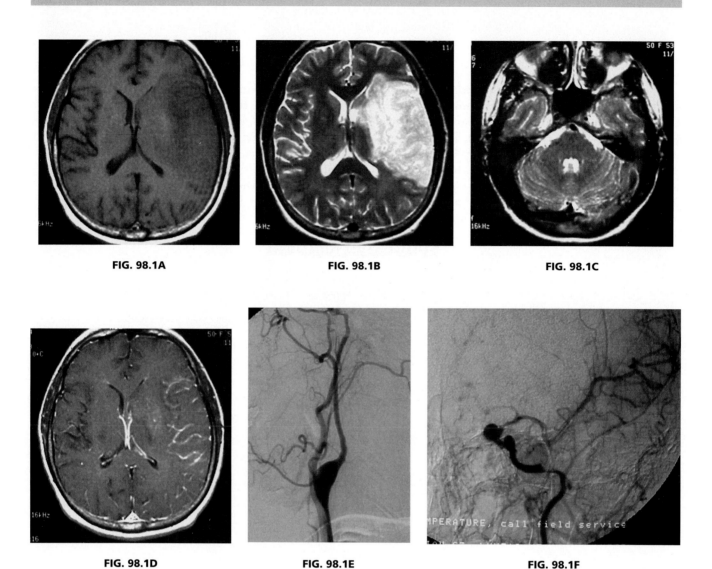

FIG. 98.1A **FIG. 98.1B** **FIG. 98.1C**

FIG. 98.1D **FIG. 98.1E** **FIG. 98.1F**

CLINICAL HISTORY

A 50-year-old woman with sudden onset of right hemiparesis.

FINDINGS

Axial T1-weighted and T2-weighted acquisitions (Fig. 98.1A and B) demonstrate a large wedge-shaped region of signal abnormality involving the cortex and subcortical white matter of the left frontal and parietal lobes in the left middle cerebral artery distribution. The region is hypointense on T1-weighted acquisition and hyperintense on T2-weighted images. There is effacement of the left lateral ventricle, as well as slight displacement of the midline structures toward the right. There is diffuse effacement of overlying cortical sulci. More inferiorly on the T2-weighted image (Fig. 98.1C), the flow void within the cavernous portion of the left internal carotid artery is significantly smaller when compared with the right. Following intravenous contrast (Fig. 98.1D), there is marked intravascular enhancement in the left middle cerebral artery territory.

DIAGNOSIS

Acute cortical infarct secondary to carotid dissection.

DISCUSSION

Most strokes are ischemic in origin (90%) while the rest are hemorrhagic. Ischemic stroke can be caused by emboli from distant sites, such as the heart or proximal vessels, or can result from local vessel thrombosis. Local thrombosis typically occurs because of an inherent vessel abnormality, such as atherosclerosis, dissection (as seen in this case), or vasculitis. Large vessel occlusion accounts for most cerebral infarctions, resulting in large cortically based infarcts, which fall within the vascular territory of the involved vessel. Small vessel occlusion is usually the result of microatheroma or wall hyalinization in the setting of hypertension. Occlusion of these small vessels results in small (less than 1 cm) focal infarcts of the basal ganglia and other deep brain structures, termed "lacunar infarcts."

MRI is the most sensitive modality in the detection of early infarction. Eighty percent are visible on standard spin echo MRI obtained within 24 hours of ictus. The earliest finding of ischemia on MRI is absence of normal flow void within the vessel supplying the affected area. Slow flow within cortical vessels can be seen as intravascular enhancement on postcontrast imaging (seen in this case). Intravascular enhancement is a common finding in acute cortical infarction, seen in 75% of cases. These MRI signs can be detected within minutes of symptom onset. Brain swelling is another early finding, which is best seen on T1-weighted images. It often precedes T2-weighted hyperintensity in the affected area, which may be seen within 1 to 2 hours but may take 8 hours to develop following symptom onset. In approximately one third of cases, abnormal meningeal enhancement can be seen along the involved cortex. In 10% to 20% of acute infarction, standard MRI will be normal.

As infarction progresses into the subacute stage (after the first 24 to 48 hours), the intravascular and meningeal enhancement begins to diminish. Parenchymal enhancement ensues (often a patchy gyriform pattern) and can persist for 8 to 10 weeks. Edema becomes the most prominent finding at 24 to 48 hours, characterized by hypointense cortex and subcortical white matter on T1-weighted images and hyperintense signal on proton density–weighted, T2-weighted, and fluid-attenuated inversion-recovery images. Wedge-shaped signal abnormality is typically seen in large vessel cortical infarcts (shown in this case). Mass effect increases during the second and third day and then gradually decreases after 7 to 10 days. During the second week, T2-weighted hyperintensity will decrease and may disappear. This is referred to as the "fogging" effect. At this time, there

can be striking parenchymal enhancement in the involved vascular distribution with very little to no signal abnormality on T2-weighted images. The subacute phase of arterial infarction can be complicated by hemorrhagic transformation, occurring in up to 33% of large middle cerebral infarctions. Petechial hemorrhage can be seen in up to 50% of infarcts in the second to third week.

Encephalomalacia is the area of nonviable or "soft brain" left behind after a large cortical infarction. It is characterized by a well-defined area of low signal on T1-weighted images with high signal (following that of cerebrospinal fluid) on long TE acquisitions. The overlying cortical sulci and ipsilateral ventricle enlarge, reflecting loss of cerebral parenchyma. Mass effect and contrast enhancement are absent. Degeneration and atrophy of the associated axons and their myelin sheath is termed "wallerian degeneration." Linear high-signal abnormality can be seen to follow the course of the affected axons as they course from the involved cerebral cortex along the internal capsule and brainstem white matter tracts to the spinal cord.

Diffusion-weighted MRI has become the most sensitive sequence in the detection of acute infarction. Diffusion-weighted MRI is sensitive to the microscopic motion of water protons and will exhibit hyperintense signal in regions of slower proton diffusion. Cytotoxic edema is initiated within minutes of the onset of ischemia, producing a slight increase in brain-water content, shift of extracellular water into ischemic cells, resulting in diminished motion or "diffusion" of protons in affected areas. Hyperintense signal can therefore be detected on diffusion-weighted MRI within minutes of arterial occlusion.

Magnetic resonance angiography can illustrate major vessel occlusion and severe stenosis. It is less sensitive for milder degrees of stenosis and more distal lesions.

This case illustrates an acute/subacute cortical infarction in the left middle cerebral artery territory. There is wedge-shaped signal abnormality as well as intravascular enhancement. There is diminished caliber of the left cavernous portion of the carotid artery seen on MRI because of flow reduction related to dissection of the more proximal vessel. The arterial dissection of the left internal carotid artery is nicely demonstrated on the subsequent cerebral angiogram (Fig. 98.1E and F). Note abrupt smooth narrowing of the left internal carotid artery approximately 2 cm distal to the carotid bifurcation on this lateral view from a left common carotid angiogram (Fig. 98.1E). This is the classic angiographic appearance of carotid artery dissection. The left internal carotid artery is narrow and slightly irregular throughout the cervical and petrous portions of the vessel. There is an intraluminal filling defect within the petrous portion of the vessel, likely thrombus. On the oblique intracranial view (Fig. 98.1F), the intraluminal thrombus is better seen within the petrous carotid artery. Additionally, there is a saccular aneurysm arising from the supraclinoid internal carotid artery at the origin of the ophthalmic artery.

SUGGESTED READING

Asato R, Okumura R, Konishi J. Fogging effect in MR of cerebral infarct. *JCAT* 1991;15:160–162.

Fisher CM. The arterial lesions underlying lacunes. *Acta Neuropathol (Berl)* 1969;12:1.

Kunitz SC, Gross CR, Heyman A, et al. The pilot stroke data bank: definition, design and data. *Stroke* 1984;15:740.

LeBihan D, Turner R, Douek P, et al. Diffusion MR imaging: clinical applications. *AJR* 1992;159:591–599.

Lutsep HL, Albers GW, DeCraspigny A, et al. Clinical utility of diffusion-weighted magnetic resonance imaging in the assessment of ischemic stroke. *Ann Neurol* 1997;41:574–580.

Mueller DP, Yuh WTC, Fisher DJ, et al. Arterial enhancement in acute cerebral ischemia: clinical and angiographic correlation. *AJNR* 1993;14:661–668.

Osborn AG. Stroke. In: *Diagnostic neuroradiology,* 1st ed. St. Louis: Mosby, 1994:341–354.

Warach S, Li W, Ronthal M, et al. Acute cerebral ischemia: evaluation with dynamic contrast-enhanced MR imaging and MR angiography. *Radiology* 1992;182:41–47.

Yuh WTC, Crain MR, Loes DJ, et al. MR imaging of cerebral ischemia: findings in the first 24 hours. *AJNR* 1991; 12:621–629.

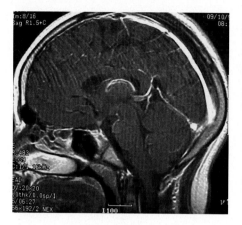

FIG. 99.1A

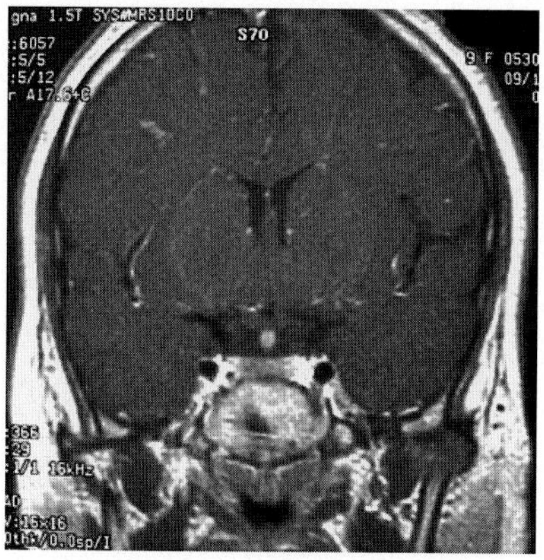

FIG. 99.1B

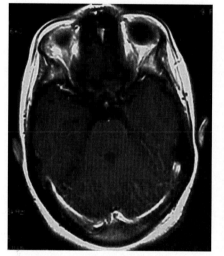

FIG. 99.1C

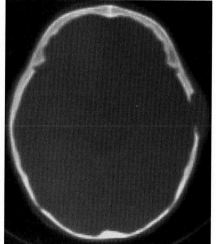

FIG. 99.1D

CLINICAL HISTORY

A 9-year-old girl with history of diabetes insipidus.

FINDINGS

Sagittal and coronal postcontrast T1-weighted acquisitions (Fig. 99.1A and B) demonstrate an enlarged enhancing infundibulum. Axial T1-weighted acquisition (Fig. 99.1C) shows that the infundibulum is larger than the basilar artery, seen as a flow void along the ventral aspect of the brainstem. The remainder of the brain was unremarkable.

DIAGNOSIS

Eosinophilic granuloma.

DISCUSSION

Eosinophilic granulomatosis or Langerhans cell histiocytosis (LCH) (formerly known as "histiocytosis X") is a disorder of the reticuloendothelial system that occasionally involves the central nervous system (CNS). Hand-Schuller-Christian syndrome is a form of LCH that occurs in early childhood and accounts for 15% to 40% of the histiocytoses. The classic triad of clinical findings includes diabetes insipidus, exophthalmos, and lytic bone lesions. CNS LCH is the result of abnormal proliferation of histiocytes (macrophages). These histiocytic granulomas most frequently involve the hypothalamus, pituitary stalk, and calvarium (as seen in this case).

Classic imaging features include marked thickening of the infundibulum with or without involvement of the hypothalamus. There is striking enhancement following contrast on both CT and MRI. In those patients with overt diabetes insipidus, the posterior pituitary "bright spot" is often absent. The infundibulum is considered enlarged when the diameter is greater than 2.5 mm. A useful rule of thumb is that the normal diameter of the infundibulum is always smaller than that of the adjacent basilar artery.

Rarely, LCH can involve other regions of the brain parenchyma with diffuse regions of prolonged T1 and T2 signal primarily involving the brainstem and cerebellum. Scattered punctate lesions throughout the cerebrum have also been described. Lesions markedly enhance following contrast. Dural disease has also been reported.

An enlarged infundibulum is a nonspecific neuroimaging finding with an extensive differential diagnosis. The differential for an infundibular mass in a child includes LCH, germinoma, and meningitis. Less common possibilities include lymphoma, glioma, and tuberculosis. In adults, the differential includes sarcoidosis, germinoma, metastasis, lymphoma, glioma, tuberculosis, and choristoma.

A search for additional imaging findings can help narrow the differential possibilities. In LCH, identification of the typical lytic calvarial lesions (seen on an axial CT scan of the brain in this case [Fig. 99.1D]) can clinch the diagnosis.

LCH calvarial lesions are well-defined lytic lesions centered within the outer table on the calvarium. The differential involvement of the inner and outer table creates the typical "beveled edge" appearance, nicely seen on this CT scan. There is typically no internal matrix or peripheral sclerosis. A central button sequestrum may be identified. The associated soft tissue mass is usually isointense with brain on T1-weighted images and heterogeneously hyperintense on T2-weighted images. There is intense enhancement following contrast, occasionally a dural "tail" of enhancement is seen along the adjacent galea or temporal muscle.

SUGGESTED READING

Maghnie M, Arico M, Villa A, et al. MR of the hypothalamic-pituitary axis in Langerhans cell histiocytosis. *AJNR* 1992;13(5):1,365–1,371.

Osborn AG. Brain tumors and tumorlike masses: classification and differential diagnosis. In: *Diagnostic neuroradiology*, 1st ed. St. Louis: Mosby, 1994:482.

Rosenfield NS, Abrahams J, Komp D. Brain MR in patients with Langerhans cell histiocytosis: findings and enhancement with Gd-DTPA. *Pediatr Radiol* 1990;20:433–436.

Schmitts S, Wichmann W, Martin E, et al. Pituitary stalk thickening with diabetes insipidus preceding typical manifestations of Langerhans cell histiocytosis in children. *Eur J Pediatr* 1993;152(5):399–401.

Tien RD, Newton TH, McDermott MW, et al. Thickened pituitary stalk on MR images in patients with diabetes insipidus and Langerhans cell histiocytosis. *AJNR* 1990;11:703–708.

Vourtsi A, Papadopoulos A, Moulopoulos LA, et al. Langerhans cell histiocytosis with involvement of the pons: case report. *Neuroradiology* 1998;40(3):161–163.

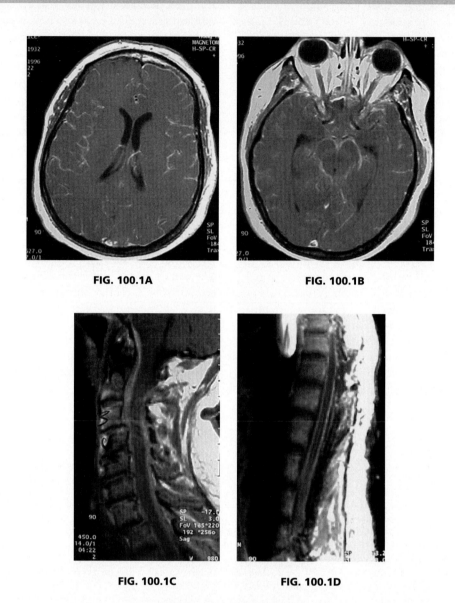

FIG. 100.1A

FIG. 100.1B

FIG. 100.1C

FIG. 100.1D

CLINICAL HISTORY

A 72-year-old woman presents with severe headache following recent dental surgery.

FINDINGS

Axial postcontrast T1-weighted acquisitions (Fig. 100.1A and B) demonstrate meningeal enhancement, as well as enhancement throughout the basal cisterns. Sagittal postcontrast T1-weighted image through the craniovertebral junction and cervical spine demonstrates thick leptomeningeal enhancement along the dorsal and ventral aspect of the spinal cord (Fig. 100.1C and D).

DIAGNOSIS

Staphylococcal meningitis, subdural empyema.

DISCUSSION

Acute meningitis may be difficult to detect with either CT or brain MRI scanning, as there may be insufficient hyperemia of the meninges to demonstrate enhancement. In this case, fulminant meningitis resulted from a subdural empyema extending throughout the spinal canal in this patient who was immunocompromised due to hypogamma-globulinemia, presumably due to hematogenous spread of infection following dental work 1 week previously.

Acute meningitis may require lumbar puncture for defini-tive diagnosis. The fluid-attenuated inversion-recovery imaging sequence can be helpful (not available in this case) by showing the proteinaceous nature of the spinal fluid in the meningeally lined sulci and its resulting increase in signal intensity. Neurological evaluation of this patient revealed diffuse paresis and obtundation, which rapidly progressed into delirium and the semicomatose state. Rapid institution of intravenous antibiotics prevented death and allowed a very slow but incomplete recovery of neurological status.

SUGGESTED READING

Mathews VP, Kuharik MA, Edwards MK, et al. Dyke Award. Gd-DTPA-enhanced MR imaging of experimental bacterial meningitis: evaluation and comparison with CT. *AJR* 1989;152(1):131–136.

Runge VM, Wells JW, Williams NM, et al. Detectability of early brain meningitis with magnetic resonance imaging. *Invest Radiol* 1995;30(8):484–495.

Sze G, Zimmerman RD. The magnetic resonance imaging of infectious and inflammatory diseases. *Radiol Clin North Am* 1988;26:839–859.

SUBJECT INDEX

W

Wallerian degeneration, 213
Watershed infarct, of cerebral arteries,
    58–59, 58f
Weakness
    left-sided
        in tumefactive acute disseminated
            encephalomyelitis, 76
        in watershed infarct of cerebral arteries,
            58–59
    lower extremities
        in meningioma of foramen magnum,
            126
        in multiple sclerosis, 78
    right-sided
        after basal ganglia infarct, 30–31
        in arteriovenous malformation, 174
        in malignant ependymoma, 132
Wernicke encephalopathy, vs. Leigh disease,
    197
White matter
    lobar, diffuse axonal injury of, 21
    radiation necrosis of, 29

X

Xanthoastrocytoma, pleomorphic, 138–139,
    138f

Y

Yolk sac tumors, 161